# *breast* implants

## *everything you need to know*

THIRD EDITION

# Nancy Bruning

Hunter House
PUBLISHERS

Hunter House Inc., Publishers
PO Box 2914
Alameda CA 94501-0914

Acknowledgment is made for permission to reprint photographs of reconstruction surgery performed by Stephen S. Kroll, M.D., Houston, Texas, pp. 49, 53, 59; photographs of augmentation and reconstruction surgeries performed by Loren Eskenazi, M.D., San Francisco, California, pp. 45, 56, 57, 139, 155. Photograph of saline implants on p. 40 courtesy of McGhan; illustrations on pp. 47, 52, 55, and 125 courtesy of National Cancer Institute; photographs of silicone in the body on pp. 94 and 95 courtesy of Rahim Karjoo, M.D.; mammograms p. 84 and diagram on p. 129 courtesy of Melvin Silverstein, M.D. Illustrations on pp. 44 and 46 © 1992 by Fran Milner. Photographs on pp. 70, 72, and 137 by Anne Stansell, Photographer ©.

*Library of Congress Cataloging-in-Publication Data*

<u>is available</u>

*Project Credits*
Cover Design & Production: Lesli Wuco-B, Jil Weil
Book Production: Hunter House
Copy Editor: Kelley Blewster
Proofreader: Rachel E. Bernstein
Indexer: Nancy D. Peterson
Acquisitions Editor: Jeanne Brondino
Associate Editor: Alexandra Mummery
Publicity Coordinator: Earlita K. Chenault
Customer Service Manager: Christina Sverdrup
Order Fulfillment: Lakdhon Lama
Administrator: Theresa Nelson
Computer Support: Peter Eichelberger
Publisher: Kiran S. Rana

Printed and bound by Bang Printing, Brainerd, Minnesota
Manufactured in the United States of America

9  8  7  6  5  4  3  2  1      Third Edition      02  03  04  05  06

# Breast Implants

## Everything You Need to Know

"*Breast Implants: Everything You Need to Know* is an unbiased presentation of information for health-care professionals and women throughout the United States. As a best-selling health writer, Ms. Bruning brings together her extensive research in this one book, and writes in a manner that is easily understandable by all women. It is complete, yet not overwhelming to the reader. The book provides answers to many of our questions about breast implants. It will help address many of our uncertainties and will help us to control our fears. By providing guidelines and direction for the future, Ms. Bruning's book serves as a vital resource for women, their families, and loved ones."

*— Amy R. Niles, Executive Director,*
*National Women's Health Resource Center*

"Nancy Bruning's *Breast Implants* helps sort out the complicated issues surrounding breast implants. The author presents the latest information in a clear and sensitive style. She covers everything from the history of implants to the surgical procedures involved to what women can do if something goes wrong. Bruning reveals the newest research about silicone disease, and clearly defines all the options, especially those not involving implants. I highly recommend this book."

*— Jenny Jones, Talk Show Host*

"[T]his book is part of the ongoing revolution in women's health care, since it presents women with the information they need to assess the situation in light of their own lives and make informed choices for the future."

*— CAREER WOMAN*

"Ms. Bruning has done a good job of identifying many key issues for women facing questions about breast implants.... [She] has nicely laid out a chapter on decision-making about implants; this information is likely to be quite helpful to women facing the dilemma of whether or not to have reconstruction or augmentation of the breast. The section on resources and the bibliography are thorough and well organized. The diagrams and other illustrations are clear and easy to interpret."

*— Journal of the National Cancer Institute*

"*Breast Implants: Everything You Need to Know*... contains the latest information from consumer health advocates, the FDA and the medical community."
*— Y-ME Hotline*

"[Bruning's] excellent book answers all the questions for which we have answers at this time in a straightforward style that will be easy for lay readers to understand....An excellent bibliography and list of information and support organizations are appended. Highly recommended for public libraries."
*— LIBRARY JOURNAL*

"This timely book provides a well-balanced view of the controversy surrounding its subject."
*— BOOKLIST*

"Discussions of reconstruction options, personal experiences, and warning signs of implant problems make for an informative guide."
*— THE MIDWEST BOOK REVIEW*

"*Breast Implants*... is a complete source of information on the subject examining all the information that is currently available about breast implants....[It] provides vital information for women when they need it most."
*— WISCONSIN BOOKWATCH*

# Other books by Nancy Bruning

*The Real Vitamin and Mineral Book* (with Shari Lieberman, Ph.D.)

*Coping with Chemotherapy*

*Dare to Lose* (with Shari Lieberman, Ph.D.)

*Female and Forgetful* (with Dr. Elisa Lottor)

*Rhythms and Cycles: Sacred Patterns in Everyday Life*

*Methylation Miracle* (with Paul Frankel, Ph.D.)

*Effortless Beauty: 10 Steps to Inner and Outer Radiance the Ayurvedic Way* (with Dr. Helen Thomas)

*Natural Relief for Your Child's Asthma: A Guide to Controlling Symptoms and Reducing Your Child's Dependence on Drugs* (with Steven Bock, M.D., and Kenneth Bock, M.D.)

*Natural Remedies for Colds and Flu*

*Ayurveda: The A–Z Guide to Healing Techniques from Ancient India* (with Dr. Helen Thomas)

*Natural Medicine for Menopause* (with Paula Maas, D.O., M.D. (H))

*Healing Homeopathic Remedies* (with Corey Weinstein, M.D.)

*The Natural Health Guide to Antioxidants: Using Vitamins and Other Supplements to Fight Disease, Boost Immunity, and Maintain Optimal Health*

*Swimming for Total Fitness* (with Jane Katz, Ed.D.)

*What You Can Do about Incontinence*

*What You Can Do about Hair Loss*

*Consultation with Your Psychotherapist* (with Elliott Seligman, Ph.D.)

*A Consumer's Guide to Contact Lenses* (with Spencer Sherman, M.D.)

*The Beach Book*

*Ordering*

Trade bookstores in the U.S. and Canada please contact:

Publishers Group West
1700 Fourth Street, Berkeley CA 94710
Phone: (800) 788-3123     Fax: (510) 528-3444

Hunter House books are available at bulk discounts for textbook course adoptions; to qualifying community, health-care, and government organizations; and for special promotions and fund-raising. For details please contact:

Special Sales Department
Hunter House Inc., PO Box 2914, Alameda CA 94501-0914
Phone: (510) 865-5282     Fax: (510) 865-4295
E-mail: ordering@hunterhouse.com

Individuals can order our books from most bookstores, by calling **(800) 266-5592**, or from our **website at www.hunterhouse.com**

# Contents

# Important Notice

The material in this book is intended to provide a review of information and resources regarding breast implants and breast-enhancing and reconstructive procedures alternative to implants. Every effort has been made to provide accurate and dependable information, and an unbiased and thorough overview of what is a controversial and at this point often speculative medical issue. The contents of this book have been compiled from interviews with medical doctors, scientists, patients, and from professional research. However, health-care professionals have differing opinions, and advances in medical and scientific research are made very quickly, so some of the information may become outdated.

Therefore, the publisher, author, and editors, and the professionals quoted in the book cannot be held responsible for any error, omission, or dated material. Any of the treatments described should be undertaken only under the guidance of a licensed health-care practitioner. The author and publisher assume no responsibility for any outcome of the use of any of these treatments in a program of self-care or under the care of a licensed practitioner.

If you have a question concerning your care or treatment, or about the appropriateness or application of the treatments described in this book, consult a health-care professional.

# Foreword

This newly revised publication of Nancy Bruning's book *Breast Implants: Everything You Need to Know* is an excellent resource for women who have implants (and their family members) as well as women who are considering implants. It carefully navigates the reader between what is known and what is not known, providing up-to-date research findings as well as a wide range of opinions from patients, physicians, the Food and Drug Administration (FDA), and other experts.

The history of breast implants is a saga of promises and broken promises, reassurances and warnings, speculation disguised as facts, and wishful thinking disguised as truth. Women have not been well-served by the media coverage, which has tended to swing from one extreme (a great option for women!) to the other (a time bomb in your breasts!) to another (women who say their implants made them sick are greedy ambulance chasers!) and only rarely capturing the distressing story of women who underwent surgery with a product that they thought was safe, only to find out that no objective studies of women with implants had ever been conducted. It seems that every pundit has an opinion about breast implants, whether or not they have ever read any of the research. As a result, the saga is made even more complex by a jumble of information and misinformation about local complications, diseases, and rupture rates. Wading through this morass, Nancy Bruning has courageously and carefully gathered information and opinions and provided it in a book that will help the approximately two million women with implants, as well as the many other men and women who care about them.

I first became involved in this saga in 1990 as a Congressional staffer, working for the House of Representatives subcommittee that oversees the FDA. I was contacted by a Senate staffer, whose mother had terrible complications as a result of breast reconstruction with silicone gel implants. I spoke to her mother, Sybil Goldrich, and other women with implants who implored us to find out if implants were really safe. But, when our chairman, Rep. Ted Weiss, asked the FDA for all the evidence they had about the safety of breast implants, we learned that the FDA had never required the manufacturers to prove that implants were safe. In our subsequent hearing and investigation, we learned that the FDA did not know whether any safety studies of women with implants had ever been conducted. We also learned that scientists at the FDA had expressed concerns about the safety of breast implants for years and had urged that studies be required, but their concerns were ignored.

Now, as the president of a nonprofit organization that uses research information to advocate for programs and policies that improve the health and well-being of women and families, I once again find myself examining all the research on breast implants. And once again, I wonder how it is that so little objective information is available about the long-term safety of a product that is sold to more than 200,000 women each year. We know more about short-term safety and complications than we did in 1990, but, unfortunately, the strongly held opinions of the many "experts" on this issue often go well beyond the facts that are available.

The opinions and statements included in this book accurately represent the available information and diversity of views on the safety of breast implants. There are no clear answers to many of the questions regarding breast implants, because more than a million women had breast implants before any objective research was conducted on women. Although several major research studies have been conducted in recent years, these studies cannot answer all the questions about the safety of breast implants because there are so many different kinds of implants in women across the country, and many of these implants are no longer on the market. The studies that were conducted are also flawed because they studied too few women who had implants for too short a period of time to evaluate long-term safety. In order to meaningfully study the long-term health risks of implants, we need research on many thousands of women who had implants for at least ten to fifteen years. That is the kind of information that women who have implants or are considering implants deserve, but that is not yet available to them.

As a breast cancer survivor, Nancy Bruning is especially sensitive to the needs of women who chose or are considering implants after a mastectomy. Unfortunately, there are even fewer studies of mastectomy patients with implants than there are of augmentation patients. Ms. Bruning meets this challenge, answering questions whenever possible, and in other cases describing opinions, experiences, and information but making it clear that we don't know as much as we should.

Women can be wise consumers when they have accurate, unbiased information. When information is incomplete, they need to rely on the best information available. Consumers can thank Nancy Bruning for putting an enormous amount of information together in a readable, informative, and empowering book.

*Diana Zuckerman, Ph.D.*
*President, National Center for Policy Research (CPR)*
*for Women & Families*

# Preface to the Third Edition

As we go to press, it is nearly ten years since the first edition of this book was published, and six years since the second. With each edition, I hope to be more hopeful about the implant situation. Each time, I am not. Although I have had my silicone-gel implant removed and replaced with a saline one and worry less, I still don't feel as confident as I'd like to be. My life still feels like the old joke in which a guy is falling through space from the roof of a tall building. As he passes each floor, someone asks him, "How's it going?" To which he invariably replies, "So far, so good."

The difference between me and this joke is, I'm not alone—there are plenty of other women in free fall, and others who have already hit the ground. The problem is, those who choose to step off the roof into a life with implants are unaware that they may be in for a rather hard landing. And that's no laughing matter. Although the media circus surrounding this issue has calmed down, the crisis is not over. The number of women and teenagers opting to have implants to increase the size of their breasts has doubled since 1997 and is now over two hundred thousand each year. Another eighty thousand women each year choose implants for breast reconstruction. Many women remain unaware that implants have still not been proven safe for either the short term or the long term. At the very least, any woman who chooses to have breast implants may be setting herself up for years of additional surgeries, whether she is among the large group of women who suffer from complications or not.

For years I have read new reports and studies, listened to scientific theories, heard the questions of the "worried well," and sympathized with the heartrending stories of desperate and suffering women. The U.S. government and the United Kingdom have both issued official reports that the plastic-surgery industry has chosen to interpret as saying that implants are safe. In actuality, what the reports conclude is that in many ways they are not safe—and in other ways we lack sufficient evidence to say one way or the other. Interestingly, the United Kingdom has recently decided to provide the public with more information than it used to about the risks of breast implants and has started a registry.

In the meantime, I continue to wonder: What's really going on here? How many women are sick because of their implants? Who is most at risk of becoming ill from implants? Will I one day fall splat to the ground and end up disabled, in a wheelchair, with a foggy brain, too? If, after all this research, I am still uncertain, how confused must the average person feel? In researching this book, I have traveled from the larger-than-life world of Barbie as plastic role model to the microscopic world of silicone as plastic molecule. I have pored over scores of medical journals and received twenty-seven-page faxes at midnight. I have gone through hundreds of pages of government reports. I have listened to ill and angry women who are convinced that implants are at the bottom of their medical problems and are committed to doing something about it. I am touched and awed by their fierce combination of outrage, energy, tenacity, and selfless dedication to providing support and information to others in spite of their pain, memory loss, and depleted finances. I have talked to scientists who are just as convinced of silicone's harmful effects and whose work is still dismissed by critics but who carry on despite the lack of peer support. I have talked with medical doctors and plastic surgeons who once were skeptical but are now less sure that silicone is as inert and biochemically compatible as we once thought. There are simply too many sick women passing through their offices. And I have heard about shoddy science and questionable medical and legal practices by people who continue to prey on women who, because of a lack of information, are vulnerable to their seductive songs.

The breast implant is—and will continue to be—"the most controversial medical device in history," according to one researcher I interviewed. We still have no consensus on the nature or extent of the illnesses caused by silicone, and we have no proven treatment except, possibly, to take the damn things out. We have no firm answers for the hundreds of thousands of women with breast implants, most of whom appear to be free of systemic complications, but who experience far more local complications than previously thought and who may suffer more in the future.

However, we have made some progress. Instead of ignoring or belittling their patients' problems, an increasing number of physicians are at least taking their patients' complaints more seriously. Researchers are doggedly unraveling the secrets of silicone–human body interaction and spinning intriguing hypotheses. Support groups have sprung up all over the country, as have Internet websites dedicated to breast-implant issues. A rather new subspecialty for lawyers is expertise in implant litigation, and there has been a global settlement of a class-action suit against implant manufacturers. Still, the subtitle of this book requires some clarification— among "everything you need to know" is first and foremost the fact that *we are still a long way from knowing everything.*

If some implant advocates seem shrill or alarmist, that is to be expected of people in free fall, with the ground rushing toward them or the taste of pavement already in their mouth. And, as a friend of mine is fond of saying, "Just because I'm acting paranoid doesn't mean they're not out to get me." Recent studies show that the silicone in breast implants does indeed migrate to other parts of the body, and that the human body does indeed react to silicone. Although the full extent of this reaction is not yet known, it is clearly time to stop telling women their problems are all in their heads, or to dismiss their concerns by saying that nothing is risk free. In this day of AIDS, Lyme disease, chronic fatigue immune deficiency, multiple chemical sensitivity, Gulf War syndrome, and Legionnaire's disease, why is the medical profession so resistant to considering that we may be seeing yet another previously unrecognized disease syndrome? When we chose to have implants to change our lives, this is not what we meant! It's not that we expect implants—or any medical device or treatment—to be risk free. Although many plastic surgeons believed the implant manufacturers and assured us that implants were safe lifetime devices, we now know there's no such thing as a free lunch. But, if it's not too much trouble, we'd like to see some prices on the menu. We may indeed still want implants, but we want to be able to decide if the benefits are worth the risks. How can we make an informed choice if we don't have the information on which to base a decision that will follow us the rest of our lives?

Recent studies from the Mayo Clinic and elsewhere are supposed to be reassuring, but the researchers themselves admit that too few women were involved to show that implants are safe. And they represent a backward way of doing scientific research (read more about this in Chapter 5). In fact, studies that have been conducted even more recently suggest that implants are not safe. This is particularly alarming in light of the fact that saline implants were officially approved by the FDA—even though, for example, 60 percent of women with saline implants have complications within four years, and one out of five requires additional surgery within three years. The FDA also recently made silicone-gel implants accessible to more women—even though almost half of women with silicone-gel implants experience a rupture within six to ten years, and in one out of five women silicone had migrated to other parts of their bodies. The late congressional representative Ted Weiss, who originally called for the breast-implant hearings, summed it up neatly when he said, "The silicone-breast-implant fiasco is a sad case of corporate indifference and regulatory mismanagement.... [T]he FDA has a critical role in assuring the safety and efficacy of medical products *before* consumers are exposed to them. After-the-fact regulation serves no one well, and should never be allowed to happen again."

*Nancy Bruning*
*May 2002*

# Acknowledgments

I would like to thank the following people for so graciously contributing their time, their thoughts, and their expertise:

Barbara Carter, R.N., D.N.S.C., consultant specialist in psychosocial issues relating to cancer and its treatment;

Nancy Carteron, M.D., rheumatologist and immunologist, California Pacific Medical Center;

Loren Eskenazi, M.D., plastic and reconstructive surgeon, California Pacific Medical Center;

Sharon Green, former executive director of Y-ME;

Libby Gross, American Cancer Society patient educator;

Neal Handel, M.D., assistant clinical professor, Division of Plastic Surgery, UCLA School of Medicine;

Richard Jobe, M.D., clinical professor of surgery, Stanford University Medical Center;

Edward Knowlton, M.D., chief of plastic surgery, John Muir Medical Center;

Susan Kolb, M.D., FACS, plastic surgeon and holistic physician, PLASTIKOS Plastic Surgery, Atlanta, Georgia;

Michael Middleton, Ph.D., M.D., assistant professor of radiology, University of California, San Diego;

Cindy Pearson, program director of the National Women's Health Network;

Saul Puszkin, Ph.D., immunopathologist, Mount Sinai School of Medicine;

Monona Rossol, industrial chemist and hygienist specializing in silicones;

Harry Spiera, M.D., chief of the division of rheumatology and clinical professor of medicine, Mount Sinai Medical Center;

Melvin Spira, M.D., professor of surgery, Division of Plastic Surgery, Baylor College of Medicine, Houston, Texas, and past president of the American Association of Plastic Surgeons;

Paul Striker, M.D., plastic surgeon in private practice, and senior attending surgeon, New York Eye and Ear Infirmary;

Diana Zuckerman, Ph.D., president of the National Center for Policy Research for Women & Families.

I am also grateful for the contributions and support of Jane Parish, patient advocate; the Planetree Health Resource Center; Jean Craig, founder and director of Cen-Tex Silicone Support, Inc.; Ilena Rosenthal, director of the Humantics Foundation for Women, based in San Diego; Kathy Keithley Johnston, Toxic Discovery Network; Catherine Cordone; Patricia Darman; Sheila Miller; Sharyn Higdon Jones, licensed counselor; Linda R. Thompson, cofounder of Project Impact; Janie Cruise, cofounder of *Silicone Scene*; Trudy Bly; Lynn Lynch; Karen Powers; Linda Dackman, author of *Up Front: Sex and the Post-Mastectomy Woman*; Victoria Wells, cofounder of *The Cancer Support Community*; fellow journalist Cathy Baron; Michael Ross; Carolie Tarble, prosthesis fitter; Patricia Warren and Kathleen Enright, friends and assistants; Marlene Mersch, research assistant; editors Jackie Melvin, Mali Apple, and Kelley Blewster; and to Hunter House, who saw the need for this book and made it actually happen.

## DEDICATION

I would like to dedicate this book to all the women whose lives are affected for better or worse by breast implants and to the physicians, researchers, and patient advocates who are dedicated to providing them with the truth and the best of care.

# Introduction

In 1980, at the age of thirty-one, I found myself living a nightmare. Still groggy from the anesthesia of a breast biopsy, I saw my surgeon's face as only a blur. But his words rang out loud and clear: "I'm afraid we've found cancer. We need to remove your breast to save your life." In the very next breath he also said, "But we're doing wonderful things with reconstruction these days. We can give you back your breast."

Although I was already familiar with breast reconstruction because I had edited a book on plastic surgery some years earlier, I found his words to be more than a comfort—they were a beacon in the frighteningly dark tunnel I had suddenly entered. The mutilation I was about to undergo could be repaired. As I reluctantly signed the consent form for the mastectomy, I clung to the thought that I would have a breast again. I continued to cling to the thought as they wheeled me to surgery the next day, and several days later as I faced the scar on my chest where my breast had been. The thought helped sustain me through nine months of chemotherapy, my recuperation afterward, and my search for the best plastic surgeon I could find.

A woman who has had breast cancer is never free from worry about a recurrence of the cancer, but implant surgery did not seem to be a health concern at the time. On the contrary, it was going to help me feel healthier emotionally. Once the surgery was performed, I thought, it would be over and done with, and I could get on with my life. And this was the case for a long time. I was relatively happy with my silicone implant and my life. I looked relatively normal. I felt healthy, was happily married, physically active, and loved the work I was doing.

But gradually, stories about silicone-implant problems and questions about their safety began to surface. Almost ten years after my implant surgery, I found myself living another nightmare, caused not by breast cancer, but by the uncertainties surrounding a medical treatment that was supposed to make me feel better, not worse.

Had I and thousands of other breast cancer survivors traded killer breasts for killer implants? Had thousands of other women who had implants to increase the size of their breasts risked their health, perhaps their lives, to conform to our society's standards of beauty? How dangerous were implants, really? Was this all much ado about nothing? How did it happen that after being available for over thirty years, silicone-gel implants were now the focus of such attention? And what on earth should I do about the implant that had helped me feel whole again, that had become a part of me, but that now was causing me to lose sleep at night? The implant that, meant as a remedy, was now serving instead as a constant reminder of breast cancer?

I read everything I could get my hands on. I talked to other women who had implants or were considering them (two of these were close friends, both of whom had recently been diagnosed with breast cancer). I wrote a story about the controversy for the newsletter published by Breast Cancer Action. Just at the time the Food and Drug Administration's advisory panel made its recommendations, an editor from Hunter House called to ask if I would be interested in writing a book on the subject.

The result of that phone call is the book you hold in your hands. Because the story continues to unfold, this book doesn't contain all the answers, but it does provide the latest information based on published medical studies and reports, the FDA investigation, the latest government reports, interviews with physicians and scientists, and interviews with women who have been living with implants or their alternatives.

As such, this book is also a part of the ongoing revolution in women's health care. Too often, women's health issues are controlled by forces that are not necessarily sensitive to women's real needs and wants. Women are becoming less and less content to be told what's best for them or to stand idly by while funding goes elsewhere. We are distrustful of a system that has a history of performing unnecessary hysterectomies and cesarean sections, of stalling a major study of dietary links with breast cancer, and of limiting major studies on heart disease to men only because including women would be "too complicated." More and more we are turning to each other for information and support and demanding better treatment from the regulatory and medical powers that be.

The breast-implant controversy is also part of a larger issue that affects all of us—women, men, young, old. As breast-implant activist Linda Thompson said to me:

> Corporations can do whatever they want to. In his book *In the Absence of the Sacred* Jerry Mander says that corporations have no souls; there's no one individual in charge. This applies to what we're seeing here, and to many other dangerous products. The FDA is not doing its job, and because of political pressure it probably won't do its job. It's up to us—the grassroots consumers. You can't listen to these women, you can't hear similar stories over and over again and think it's only 1 percent that's sick. And even if it is only 1 percent of women with implants that are affected, why not take care of that 1 percent? Why do they continue to meet with denial, and why are they looked at as if they weren't there?

Unfortunately, we still have a long way to go. An estimated one to two million women already have implants, and last year another three hundred thousand women had implant surgery. Twice as many teenagers are getting implants as got them three years ago. They are doing this because they believe implants will improve their quality of life. Yet the vast majority of studies conclusively show that for many women, implants reduce quality of life and thrust them on a merry-go-round of complications, more surgery, scarring, and deformity. And other studies suggest serious health consequences, such as an increase in certain types of cancer, respiratory illness, suicide, autoimmune disease, as well as difficulty diagnosing breast cancer.

Even if you believe you are one of the lucky ones, your implants will not last forever, and in all likelihood you will need to have your implants removed and replaced at least every fifteen years or so. This alone should cause you to pause. As one recipient of implants for cosmetic reasons told me, "When I got my silicone implants there wasn't much controversy, and to tell the truth I was more concerned about the cosmetic results anyway. I'm not really concerned about the controversy now—I don't even think about it. But they never really told us that we'd need to replace them at some point, did they?"

I have two hopes. The first is that this book encourages all women who have implants or are considering them to seize control of their lives and get the information they need to make the best decision for themselves at this time. What do we know now about the health risks of implants? How do you recognize the warning signs? What should you do if you have an implant and feel you are in danger? How do you make a decision about having breast reconstruction or augmentation—and what are your options besides implants?

My second hope is that in the not too distant future we will have the information we desperately need that will allow us either to live comfortably with implants, to have available safer implants, or to take specific action to live without them.

If both of these hopes become reality, then—as painful as it has been—the controversy surrounding breast implants will have served a very useful purpose.

# 1

# The Story Unfolds

Whether you are considering getting breast implants, or already have implants and are wondering what to do about them, you might be surprised to learn that breast implants have not been thoroughly tested for safety, and until recently none of them were ever actually approved by the Food and Drug Administration (FDA). In 2000, the FDA officially approved saline-filled implants made by two companies for general use, but many scientists and women's health advocates believe the implants have not been studied thoroughly enough to warrant government approval. For saline- and silicone-gel-filled implants alike, the questions remain: How could women's doctors, whom the women trusted, put something in their bodies that had not actually been proven safe, in neither the short term nor the long term? How did it happen that the regulatory system established to protect us became the focus of what has been dubbed "the implant circus"?

Although the circus has folded its tent, there is still a very large gorilla in the room. The gorilla is the question of safety, but the media chooses to ignore it. Instead of covering the health risks of silicone implants and interviewing women with implants as it did in the early days of the controversy, it has switched its focus to the financial concerns of the implant manufacturers and medical industry.

If you are a current or potential breast-implant "consumer" you have some tough decisions ahead of you. I think the first step in making those decisions is to understand something about the still-unfolding history of breast implants and how we got to this point. It's a story of widely differing motivations, emotional reactions, and opinions among all the players involved: the FDA, the implant manufacturers, the plastic surgeons and other physicians, the attorneys, the consumer-advocate groups, and the millions of women who are caught in the middle—and that means you.

## The History of Silicone

Silicone is a synthetic plastic, or polymer, that was first developed in the 1930s. It is made from silicon, a metal-like substance found in nature that when combined with oxygen forms silica. Ordinary beach sand, crystals, and quartz are really silica. When silica is combined with carbon, it forms silicon, and when this is further processed, it becomes polymerized, a process in which simple molecules are combined to form more complex molecules. This polymerized silicon is silicone.

Silicone can be processed into three forms: a fluid, a gel, and a solid rubberlike compound known as an elastomer. In its various forms, silicone has been used for medical purposes for over sixty years. It has been used in artificial joints, pacemakers, artificial heart valves, hypodermic needles, penile and testicular implants, various kinds of tubes, drains, and catheters, lenses used in the eyes, and as a lubricant. Silicone is also used in many items you find around the house—polishes, suntan and hand lotions, antiperspirants, soaps, processed foods, waterproof coatings, chewing gum—even baby formulas and certain nonprescription drugs that aid digestion.

In the late 1940s, physicians began to inject silicone liquid directly into the body to fill out certain parts, including the face to smooth out wrinkles and the breasts to make them larger. But injecting large amounts of silicone caused problems in some women. Some women even died from the injections. Using silicone for this purpose was eventually banned, although some physicians continued the practice.

Early breast implants were made of polyurethane foam, paraffin, steel, and grafts of human tissue. These were unsuccessful, and when the first silicone breast implants became available in the early 1960s, they were hailed as a breakthrough. Although an improvement over the earlier materials, the first silicone implants had problems as well. They were firm, and therefore surgeons were required to make several large surgical incisions to insert them, a practice that often left women with prominent scars.

Gradually, the product improved. With the advent of thinner silicone gel, implants felt softer and looked more natural. They were also quite pliable, so they could be inserted using much smaller incisions.

Before the FDA ruling in 1992 (see page 12), several types of implants were available to all women: silicone-gel-filled implants (the most frequently used type), saline-filled implants, and double-lumen implants (a combination of silicone gel and saline). These are described in greater detail in Chapter 3.

## The FDA Enters the Scene

Although breast implants had been available since the early 1960s, it was not until 1976 that Congress gave the FDA authority to regulate implants and other medical devices. At that point breast implants had been in use for some time, so they were simply "grandfathered." This means they were allowed to remain on the market, even though they had not been subjected to the stringent testing required before approval of brand-new products.

Many other devices and medications were similarly grandfathered (for example, culture mediums, catheters, pacemaker components, dental materials used in fillings and root canals, the artificial larynx, surgical materials, and artificial eyes), because the FDA felt there was no evidence that they were harmful. The agency's decision was based on the premise that, in general, more is known about the safety of a device that has been in use for some time than about one that is newly developed. The law also gave the FDA authority to go back and require that the manufacturers provide proof that the implants were indeed safe and effective, if it believed there was reason to do so. However, it took the FDA a very long time to decide to take this step.

## Implants Get a New Classification

Manufacturers were aware that silicone from implants could "bleed" through the envelope and migrate to other parts of the body. However, it was widely believed that pure, medical-grade silicone was inert, chemically and physically stable during contact with body tissues, did not cause inflammation, was nonallergenic, and had no adverse long-term effects on the body. Thus, the overriding scientific reaction to migrating silicone was: So what?

We know now that as far back as 1978, staffers at the FDA wanted to move implants to another product category—one that required more rigorous testing. The FDA commissioner at that time rejected the idea. However, reports of problems with silicone-gel-filled breast implants—including leaking and rupture, inflammation, and hardening of the breasts—became too numerous to ignore.

By 1982, the FDA had received thousands of such complaints and finally moved the devices to Class III, a more stringent category that requires manufacturers to supply scientific evidence to prove the products are safe, even while leaving them on the market. Meanwhile, reports of other adverse effects heated up the controversy. These included allegations of autoimmune diseases such as rheumatoid arthritis, scleroderma, and lupus erythematosus. Six years later, in 1988, the FDA issued final regulations regarding the reclassification and required manufacturers to submit safety data within thirty months. While the public waited, implants boomed in popularity, and the estimated number of women receiving implants annually climbed to over one hundred thousand.

## The Controversy Heats Up

In 1990, Representative Ted Weiss, chairman of the House Subcommittee on Human Resources and Intergovernmental Relations that oversees the FDA, asked the FDA what was taking so long. Hearings were held, and patients and doctors testified about the health problems linked with implants. One of these patients was Sybil Goldrich, who told of body rashes, fever, pain, hardened breasts, and several surgeries to remove and replace her foam-covered implants. (Goldrich went on to form a consumer group, the Command Trust Network, and the manufacturer of her implants eventually stopped making foam-covered implants.) The hearings created a lot of sensational media coverage, and Connie Chung and "60 Minutes" both did exposés. Finally, the FDA issued a formal request for safety data within ninety days, or all silicone implants would be withdrawn from the market.

Nearly ten years after the new classification, the manufacturers submitted their data to the FDA, which had a new commissioner, David Kessler. The FDA assembled a twenty-two-member advisory panel to review the material. The panel consisted of health professionals, consumer representatives, and an industry representative. In November 1991, the advisory panel found that the data were insufficient to establish the safety of the implants and recommended that manufacturers be given more time to collect and submit data. Although concerned, at this point the FDA was insufficiently alarmed to remove the implants from the market.

Meanwhile, an increasing number of women suffering from a variety of conditions began to file lawsuits against implant manufacturers. In November 1991, a California jury awarded a landmark $7.3 million to Mariann Hopkins, who had suffered immune-system problems. Her implants had ruptured, and the jury believed her problems were due to the silicone even though her own doctors testified that her symptoms began before she received her implants. (In August 1994, the U.S. Court of Appeals upheld the $7.3 million verdict.)

The defendant, Dow Corning Wright, was found guilty of fraud and was eventually forced to release internal memos leaked from one of the implant patient trials. These were very damning and showed that staffers at Dow Corning Wright, the largest manufacturer of silicone implants, had doubts about the product's safety as early as 1971 but that these concerns were ignored. There were implications that the company had skimped on premarket testing. "Of the 329 studies by Dow Corning, only a handful (if that many) were conducted on humans," according to Dr. Diana Zuckerman. And, she says, most were engineering studies, for example, stretching the implants to see when they would break; however, implants react differently when placed in the human body which has a temperature of 98.6 degrees Fahrenheit. Robert LeVier, a technical director at Dow, testified that the longest testing period of silicone gel before its new thin-shelled, fluid-gel implant was marketed in 1975 lasted a mere eighty days. In fact, it seemed that a Dow employee ordered the reduction of gel testing from ninety days to eighty days to be able to display the implant at trade shows and plastic-surgeon meetings before June 1975. In addition, LeVier conducted a six-month study in rabbits in 1978, using the stiffer gel used in pre-1975 implants. Even this firmer gel migrated and broke down, and LeVier concluded that humans should not be exposed to free silicone until further studies showed it was safe.

Around the time of the hearing, the American Society of Plastic and Reconstructive Surgeons (ASPRS) mounted a four-million-dollar campaign for "balanced coverage" of the issue; the money was spent on lobbying, advertising, patient education, and research. The ASPRS also conducted a letter-writing effort and brought four hundred women who were satisfied with their implants to Washington to lobby Congress.

The lawsuits, media coverage, and new information heightened the FDA's concern and created even more public hysteria. In January 1992, FDA Commissioner Kessler declared a voluntary moratorium on the distribution and use of silicone-gel implants. In addition, the advisory panel was to meet again after public hearings were held in February 1992 to decide what to do about the implants.

During the deliberation period in 1991 and 1992, the FDA received thousands of letters from women with breast implants. The majority were satisfied, but a small group (112) was not.

Among the dissatisfied group, there were four patterns of experiences:

♦ They had not received enough information before surgery

♦ They were not taken seriously by their doctors when they complained about pain or other symptoms

♦ They had trouble maintaining their usual activities

♦ They had concerns about the future and lack of information

In February 1992, the FDA established a Breast Information Line; it was in operation until July 1992 and responded to forty-one thousand callers. More than 90 percent of the callers were women, and more than 70 percent had breast implants. The information specialists who took the calls reported that half the women sounded upset, sad, fearful, or worried, and a small number sounded angry. Over half said they had physical problems, many of which were associated with autoimmune disease, implant ruptures, hardening of the breasts, and infections.

## The Findings of the FDA Advisory Panel

After the February 1992 meeting, the FDA panel felt it still lacked enough information to determine whether silicone implants were safe. The members did conclude that the rupture rate may have been higher than previously thought; that rupture may go undetected in some patients; and that the implants "bleed" small amounts of silicone, but they felt it wasn't clear yet whether this was harmful. Although Dow Corning Wright conducted 329 studies and submitted thirty thousand pages of documents, we still did not know:

♦ how often saline implants leak

♦ how often implants rupture

◆ how long implants last in the body

◆ how much and how often silicone implants leak

◆ what happens to the escaped gel in the body

◆ how often women with implants suffer adverse effects

◆ to what extent implants interfere with mammography examinations

◆ whether implants increase the risk of developing cancer

◆ the relationship between breast implants and autoimmune and connective-tissue disorders

◆ the best way to detect leaks and ruptures

### The FDA's Recommendations

Because of concerns about the lack of information, on 20 February 1992, the advisory panel recommended that breast implants be restricted. On 16 April 1992, the FDA made its official decision, based on the panel's recommendations. Silicone-gel-filled implants remained available only to women who agreed to become part of clinical studies and be closely monitored. They were restricted to women who wanted breast reconstruction after breast cancer surgery, women who had silicone implants that had ruptured and who wanted them replaced, and women with breast deformities. They all had to sign an informed consent form delineating the risks and benefits of implants—something that had not previously been required. Because the FDA considered them to be less risky, saline-filled implants, on the other hand, were allowed to stay on the market and available for both reconstruction and augmentation. The FDA also required prospective (forward-looking) studies to be conducted, but these were slow in getting started, and few and far between. Eight years later the government finally published an FDA study and the two by the National Cancer Institute; these are summarized on page 23.

# A Range of Reactions

The implant controversy and the FDA's 1992 ruling received some praise and a lot of criticism, and it stirred up a fascinating stew of emotional reactions and opinions. Patients, consumer advocates, and health professionals differed widely in their reactions to what has been called the biggest medical-device controversy since the furor over the intrauterine Dalkon shield in the 1970s.

## Finally, Scientific Studies

Most agreed that it would be wise to finally have reliable scientific information about implants, which would settle the dispute as to whether they were safe and effective or not. In its response to the FDA decision, the National Women's Health Network said it was pleased that the FDA was "formally acknowledging the experimental status of silicone breast implant surgery....This communicates the serious intent of the FDA to require sound research, and to hold manufacturers and surgeons responsible for providing accurate information about breast implant risks as well as benefits." But opinions differed as to how much more we really needed to know and whether manufacturers would be able or willing to pay for definitive studies.

## The FDA Went Too Far

Some feared that because of severe restrictions and all the hoopla about possible adverse effects, silicone implants would disappear, taking a perfectly good device—one that had benefited many women—off the market. Our options would be reduced, these critics concluded, perhaps with little or no reason. Some worried that the concerns about silicone-gel implants would be "distorted" to include saline implants as well.

## The FDA Didn't Go Far Enough

While some accused the FDA of being too zealous, others accused it of stopping short of what was needed. Dr. Sidney Wolfe, of the

Public Citizen Health Research Group, was one of these. He felt it was wrong to continue what he called a thirty-year experiment with silicone gel, since there were known risks. He, and others, would rather have seen silicone implants banned completely.

## The Ruling Established a Double Standard

The FDA decision restricted gel implants for cosmetic purposes, but made them freely available to women for reconstruction because they had "a greater need." Some said this was, in essence, a double standard, and that the need to feel whole again after a mastectomy was no more valid than the desire to have implants for cosmetic reasons when we live in a culture that exerts tremendous pressure on women to be well-endowed.

Paul Striker, a plastic surgeon, was furious because "[t]he distinction between reconstruction and augmentation is totally irrational. A woman who has had breast cancer and is already injured from surgery, radiation, or chemotherapy, who may not be in the greatest health, who may have cancer cells left in her, is being allowed to have an implant which they feel is dangerous in a healthy woman." He argued that silicone implants may be even more dangerous in a woman with breast cancer.

Many breast cancer patients agreed with the woman who put it to me this way: "Oh, so this means we're expendable—we'll probably die of cancer anyway,…so let's experiment on us. It doesn't matter as much if an implant is dangerous."

## Freedom of Choice

A related issue is that of freedom of choice—who is to say that the quality of life afforded by implants is more important and greater for the woman with breast cancer than for the woman who has augmentation? "We saw the decision as sort of arrogant," says Sharon Green, executive director of the breast cancer organization Y-ME. "Some of the women who called us really had very strong, thought-out reasons for choosing augmentation. If you feel that women with breast cancer have a right to choose implants, then you must also believe that women who want implants for augmentation have an equal right to choose. To say that women should have a choice for one and not the other is inconsistent." Striker adds, "A woman should weigh the risks and benefits and make her own decision—she doesn't have to be protected from herself."

And the *Wall Street Journal* observed, "It's a strange feminism that prohibits women from choosing to decide for themselves what risks they will take." Of course, as Representative Ted Weiss pointed out, "How can women make an informed choice when there is no reliable information about risks?"

## A Moral Judgment

Norman Cole, who was at that time the president of the American Society of Plastic and Reconstructive Surgeons, said of the ruling, "The government has placed itself in the role of judging the morality of a woman's reasons for choosing implants." He argued that if silicone is considered safe for one purpose, it ought to be considered safe for the other. (We must also bear in mind that, in the past, the ASPRS has referred to small breasts as a "disease.")

Rita Freedman, who was on the FDA advisory panel, was quoted in the 9 January 1992 issue of the *Wall Street Journal* "Review and Outlook" as stating that breast reconstructions "perpetuate the myth of the Barbie Doll body." To which Jane Parish, who has had reconstruction for breast cancer and is an advocate for breast cancer patients, responded: "That is just sheer garbage! Has Rita Freedman had breast cancer? Has she ever been stared at because she only has one breast?"

Another panel member was quoted as saying that the FDA "should deliver a profoundly important message to the American public involving basic values, concepts of beauty...." I wonder: Since when is it the FDA's job to make moral judgments about the issues of beauty and breast size?

## Perpetuates Misunderstanding of Risk and Safety

We can't expect to enjoy benefits without risks. Striker, who has been using saline implants exclusively for decades, says, "Surgery is dangerous, period. No medical implant can be considered perfectly safe, or not be associated with adverse effects in a small number of patients if it is used for any meaningful length of time."

## What Went Wrong?

In the process of attempting to deal with questions about implants, the "circus" exposed weaknesses in the regulatory system and posed crucial questions for every group involved. As one plastic surgeon I spoke to said, "We've all got some skeletons in our closets." No one is completely blameless in this fiasco.

### The FDA

The FDA was criticized for looking the other way and dragging their feet. In a *Mother Jones* article, investigative reporter Nicholas Regush contended that "FDA officials bowed to the interests of plastic surgeons and manufacturers and turned their backs on the women who used breast implants." His article stated that Ted Weiss's subcommittee found that the concerns of FDA scientists were stymied by higher-level officials for years, and that the agency was crippled by the Reagan administration's deregulation policy and lack of funding.

In 1991, a federal advisory panel concluded that the FDA needed to be strengthened by providing it with more money, more staff, and improved facilities. At that time, the FDA conducted no testing on its own; it merely reviewed studies that the manufacturers conducted and paid for. Some argued that such a practice could not possibly result in well-conducted, reliable, impartial studies and that the whole testing, monitoring, and approval system needed an overhaul. (In fact, the FDA finally conducted a study in 2001, and the results were unfavorable to implants. It found that women with leaking silicone-gel implants were more likely to suffer from autoimmune and related illnesses.)

Jane Parish was one of many who were troubled by the makeup of the FDA "expert advisory panel." She asked:

> Why did the FDA dismiss three of their experts in recon-
> structive surgery from the advisory panel one week prior to

the hearing on gel breast implants? During the FDA hearing on the Silastic cataract lens, three ophthalmologists served on the advisory panel. Why the change in protocol for the breast-implant advisory panel? Half of the voting members on the breast-implant advisory panel are not scientists, reconstructive surgeons, or physicians. Yet, they will supposedly be evaluating scientific data. Why didn't the FDA invite panel members who are experts in the breast-implant field?

Edward Knowlton, chief of plastic surgery at John Muir Medical Center, was dismayed that the FDA used Dow's internal memos from the Hopkins case, calling it "[a] process that lends itself to distortion, not objective scientific analysis." And in Striker's view, "It's a sad thing that science was taken out of the process."

## The Plastic Surgeons and the ASPRS

Knowlton believes plastic surgeons must take a certain amount of responsibility for the fiasco. He says:

> We had an enormously successful medical device and we were too complacent about it. Our big mistake was that we did not establish a breast registry. If we had, we could have supplied answers to the allegations as to whether there was any statistical evidence. It would not have become a tabloid issue. We don't even know how many implants are out there. Everything is estimates.

Neal Handel, assistant clinical professor in the Division of Plastic Surgery at UCLA School of Medicine, says:

> None of us were aware as we were using these products—we had assumed that they had been appropriately tested, that some government regulatory agency was overseeing all this. Little did we know that there was really nobody watching what was going on. I don't think the majority of us really understood the process and all that has transpired. The regulatory agencies and the approval process that medical devices go through—that's not something you learn about in medical school or during your residency. Most of us didn't concern ourselves with this until the breast-implant crisis.

Striker feels part of the problem stemmed from doctors failing to be candid in telling their patients about the probable and possible adverse effects of implants. Striker also believes that the ASPRS, "in their zeal to preserve the silicone-gel implant, perpetuated the myth that saline was a far less desirable alternative." In his experience, the saline implant is a perfectly acceptable alternative, and safer.

## The Media

The media jumped on the story with relish and for the most part seemed more interested in sensationalizing the story to sell papers and boost ratings than in furthering intelligent debate. Sharon Green, executive director of Y-ME, noted, "Our constituents [breast cancer patients] have been overwhelmingly pleased with their implants and have not experienced the kinds of problems that have been focused on in the press."

## The Implant Manufacturers

The implant manufacturers took advantage of the FDA's laissez-faire attitude. Striker says, "There may have been some laxity in conducting the studies and in the physicians examining that." Knowlton says, "A lot of us are not happy with Dow Corning. I don't know if there was a deliberate cover-up, but why didn't they let us know about the concerns that surfaced in those memos? We were totally in the dark—I think there may have been a lack of ethical behavior on their part."

## The Consumer Groups

Although consumer groups may have set out to perform a service, some feel that certain groups were overzealous in their relentless persecution of implants. In the process, they may have made statements based on innuendo and hearsay. In the end, they may have done more harm than good by causing fear and hysteria and worrying many women unnecessarily.

Loren Eskenazi, a plastic surgeon in San Francisco, was concerned about the "huge hysteria" generated by the hype:

> I've heard about documentable hysterical symptoms—one
> woman woke up one morning, unable to move. She was so
> afraid that her implants were harming her health, she began
> hallucinating, she was committed to a psychiatric hospital,
> they medicated her, and she finally got better. This, by the
> way, was a computer programmer, an intelligent woman, with
> no prior history of mental imbalance. She had her implants
> removed, switched to saline, and is doing fine.

Consumer groups added to the general confusion. On the one
hand, some accused the FDA of taking too long to approve life-
saving and life-extending drugs, and pressured the agency to act
more quickly than it had in the past. On the other hand, some
criticized the FDA for allowing faulty devices and harmful or inef-
fective drugs to be marketed before all the risks were known. We
still don't have agreement among consumer advocates. In 1996, Y-
ME National Breast Cancer Organization filed a citizen's petition
with the FDA requesting that the agency ease restrictions on the
availability of silicone-gel-filled implants for women who choose
reconstruction after a mastectomy and who have other special medical needs. A few months later, the FDA received another citizen's
petition from a group of implant recipients requesting that the
agency do just the opposite, and completely revoke permission to
make silicone-gel-filled implants available to these same women.

Conflict-of-interest charges were also raised concerning the
Public Citizen Health Research Group and the FDA. One of Commissioner Kessler's senior advisors was married to a lawyer at Public Citizen, the parent organization of the Health Research Group.
This lawyer asked the FDA in 1988 to ban silicone-gel implants,
and had sponsored conferences for plaintiff lawyers, selling them
kits for $750 on how to sue implant makers. In a *Forbes* article,
several plaintiff attorneys proudly admitted to supporting the organization "overtly, covertly, in every possible way," and one of them
was quoted as saying that Ralph Nader "is our hero.... I don't

know what the dollar amounts would be [of lawyers' contributions to the Public Citizen Health Research Group], but I think it would be very large." Joan Claybrook, president of Public Citizen, denies that lawyers contributed significant funds to the Public Citizen Health Research Group: Less than 0.5 percent, or twenty thousand dollars, came from plaintiff attorneys. This may all be coincidence, but many people wonder whom the lobby groups really represent—the consumer or the funders?

## The Consumers

As a nation, we somehow have latched on to the curious notion that we can have all the benefits of technology with none of the disadvantages—a free lunch. And when something does go wrong, we want to be able to point the finger at someone or something that is clearly to blame. Thus, we work hand in hand with plaintiff attorneys.

Many of us wanted implants so badly that we did not really want to know the downside of having a foreign object surgically implanted in our bodies. We failed to ask our plastic surgeons questions and failed to listen when they informed us of the risks. While some plastic surgeons probably told their patients only what they wanted to hear, some of us heard only what we wanted to hear. Our failure was that of being human. As Parish says of breast cancer patients, reconstruction is the only "bright spot" among all the other horrific decisions they have to make. Truly, love is blind.

## Where Are We Now?

Since the FDA ruling in 1992, we have seen several large studies, some of which seem to be reassuring, and some of which clearly are not. The reassuring studies were widely reported by the media, and this has led people to believe that silicone implants are safe over the long term. In 1999, this belief was bolstered by a report from the Institute of Medicine (IOM) on the safety of silicone breast implants. The IOM report (see sidebar below) summarized and evaluated studies that were published before 1999. The report made a clear distinction between local complications and systemic health concerns. It was most clear—and most damning—about local complications, which it considered to be the primary concern about breast implants.

Although local complications had been dismissed and down-played by the plastic-surgery industry, they can be quite serious. They include scarring, asymmetry, infection, loss of sensation in

## THE IOM REPORT

In 1997, the U.S. House of Representatives asked the Federal Depart-ment of Health and Human Services to sponsor an extensive study of silicone breast implants. The Institute of Medicine (IOM) was selected to prepare the report. A thirteen-member committee—six of them women, and consisting of members of the medical, scien-tific, and educational communities experienced in radiology, women's health, neurology, oncology, silicone chemistry, rheumatology, immunology, epidemiology, internal medicine, and plastic surgery—studied and reviewed thousands of published scientific reports, selected industry reports, and presentations from the public.

The goals of the study were to produce recommendations regarding the need for further research on breast-implant safety and to pro-vide the public with information. The committee was to:

◆ analyze silicone chemistry, toxicology, and immunology

◆ describe the many forms of implants available in the past and pres-ent

◆ review the surgical complications

◆ analyze studies on the connection between breast implants and connective-tissue, rheumatic, and neurological disease, and cancer

◆ assess the effects of implants on pregnancy, breast-feeding, and children born to mothers with implants

◆ evaluate the effects of implants on mammography and other breast-imaging techniques

The committee published a 440-page report of the results of its work. To find out where to get the report or a summary of it, see the Resources section of this book.

the breast and nipple, pain, and hardness, and can require additional surgery to correct the problems. Women may lose breast tissue because the tissue dies or because it is infiltrated with silicone and must be removed surgically. Many complications result from a more fundamental occurrence, capsular contracture (see Chapter 4)—a problem that everyone agrees does occur. What we don't know is how often it occurs, how serious it is, how to treat it, who is most likely to get it, which implants are more likely to cause it, and how to avoid it. The IOM report did conclude that a large number of women with implants could expect to have complications within one year of implantation, and to undergo an additional surgery within the first five years.

The IOM report also admitted that implants do not last a lifetime—far from it. On the contrary, they will almost certainly break at some point. As a result they will need to be surgically removed and replaced, often many times over the course of a woman's life.

The report analyzed seventeen epidemiological studies of autoimmune diseases and concluded that implants *probably* do not cause a significant increase in risk for these debilitating whole-body diseases. However, many scientists and patient advocates point out that there were serious problems with the designs of these studies, and these problems threw a shadow on any optimistic interpretation. The studies were too small to effectively study the relatively rare diseases they sought to find, and too short in duration to detect diseases that may take a long time to develop. In addition, the diseases they targeted were limited to a group of "classically defined" autoimmune diseases, and they completely ignored most other diseases and "atypical" autoimmune diseases. The scientists who conducted the studies admit to their shortcomings, yet the general impression one is left with is that implants have been proven safe.

As Diana Zuckerman, Ph.D., President, National Center for Policy Research (CPR) for Women & Families observed, "The data from these studies clearly support the view that most women do not become ill from well-defined autoimmune diseases after having implants for a short period of time. However, any conclusions about the long-term safety of implants in terms of systemic disease are premature."

As further evidence that all is not rosy, we have three studies that were conducted since 1999 and which were therefore not included in the IOM report. The studies, one conducted by the FDA and two by the National Cancer Institute (NCI), were all published in 2001. They all found statistically significant increased health risks associated with implants, and raised questions about the safety of implants over the long term. One found that women with ruptured and leaking silicone-gel implants had a higher rate of several connective-tissue diseases and of fibromyalgia; another showed that women with breast implants were at a higher risk of dying from brain tumors, lung cancer, respiratory disease, and suicide; the third study found that women with breast implants had a higher incidence of cancer in general. As Dr. Diana Zuckerman points out, in the study with more deaths from certain cancers, women were compared with other plastic surgery patients, whereas in the study with the higher general cancer rate, women were compared to other women their age. She says, "those comparisons are important to mention because plastic surgery patients are healthier than the general population (because they tend to be more affluent), so that's why implant studies need to have the appropriate comparison group."

Many women are happy with their breast implants and say that the implants have improved their quality of life. I wish them well and hope they continue to do well. For others, breast implants have brought with them physical, emotional, and financial pain. Serious, legitimate concerns are giving women who have implants many sleepless nights; these women's fears may result in their choosing to undergo what could prove to be needless surgery to have their implants removed. No matter what, many women's trust in our doctors, our lawyers, and our system of checks and balances continues to erode. As usual, the patients suffer the most. If implants had been studied properly to begin with, we would be able to make decisions based on scientific information rather than on stories, anecdotes, theories, inconclusive studies, corporate memos, and gut fear. We would not be suffering from physical and psychological pain, searching for doctors who can help us, or taking implant companies to court. We would not be agonizing over whether we should get implants, or whether we should have them removed, and our quality of life would be vastly different.

In the first edition of this book, published shortly after the FDA made its final recommendations regarding silicone-gel implants, I ended this chapter by saying, "If there are no problems, we should know. If there are problems, we should know." Two years later, in the second edition, I ended it by saying, "We know there are problems. But we still do not know exactly what they are, who is at higher risk, or how to diagnose or treat them." It's now more than ten years since Representative Ted Weiss raised the alarm about breast implants. The media circus may be over, but the medical crisis is not. We have some answers, but not all. Some of the information from the new studies is reassuring; some of it is quite worrisome.

In the meantime, what are we to do? Should breast implants be banned completely, outside of clinical trials? Should all women forgo breast implants voluntarily, or if we already have them, should we all have them taken out immediately?

Well, not quite. Although some of the problems have only recently come to light, many of the problems with implants were known to a certain degree for many years. The problem with breast implants is that—for many, many reasons—we were insufficiently aware of what the risks were. This was the dark and dirty little secret of breast implants, and we all conspired to keep it. And judging by the content of media stories, the comforting reassurances of plastic surgeons, the backlog in the courts, the paralysis of medical research, and the numbers of women who continue to clamor for artificial breasts, the conspiracy continues. We deserve safer, better implants, just as we deserve safe hip and dental implants, pacemakers, and liver transplants. In this, we all have a stake, and ignoring or denying the problems serves no one.

In 1995, Dow Corning filed for Chapter 11 bankruptcy protection. In 1999, most women in the class action suit against Dow Corning accepted a settlement plan that would pay $3.2 billion to resolve claims by more than 170,000 litigants. However, the settlement has remained tied up in bankruptcy court. According to a spokesman for Dow, the company hopes to settle the matter and emerge from bankruptcy after the settlement.

# 2

# The Benefits of Implants: Who Wants Them and Why?

No one knows exactly how many women have had breast implants, or what type they have had. No national records have been kept, so we only have estimates, which vary widely. However, it is pretty much agreed that about 1.5 to 2 million women in the United States currently have breast implants; about two-thirds of them received implants to augment their breasts, and one-third of them had implants as part of breast reconstruction to replace a breast lost to surgery to treat or prevent breast cancer. A small percentage of recipients have had their breasts removed because of fibrocystic breast lumps (a noncancerous condition that requires frequent biopsies to rule out cancer), and some had asymmetrical breasts and wanted implants to even out their appearance. The reasons women have implants are as varied as the women themselves, but they all share the desire to change their particular situation and improve their quality of life.

Our relationship with breasts appears to be rather deep-seated. We call ourselves mammals, emphasizing from the get-go what distinguishes us from other animal classes: We depend on mammary glands to nurture our young—they are the real and symbolic givers

of life. It's no accident that fertility goddesses often have voluptuous or multiple breasts. Even if we do not have or want to nurse
a child, is it any wonder we would like to restore or enhance such
an intimate yet public body part?

The American Society of Plastic and Reconstructive Surgeons
(ASPRS) did a survey in 1990 of women who had breast implants.
While this survey is not scientific, it does offer some facts and figures, as well as some insights into why these women chose to have
implants and what the benefits may be.

The 592 questionnaires that were collected indicated that most
of the women were satisfied with the results of their implants and
would choose to have the surgery again. Sixty-five percent of the
women who responded had implants for cosmetic enlargement and
35 percent for reconstruction. On the average, the women had
had their implants for eight years. As an overall group:

◆ 92.5 percent said they were satisfied with their implants

◆ 82 percent said they would do it again without a doubt

◆ 16 percent said they would probably do it again

◆ 2 percent said they would definitely not do it again

## Breast Implants after Cancer or Other Surgery: Reconstruction

Breast cancer surgery is the most common reason for breast reconstruction. There are basically two surgical procedures used to treat
breast cancer. A *mastectomy* removes all the breast tissue of the
affected breast and the lymph nodes from the armpit of that side.
A *lumpectomy* removes only the lump, plus a margin of breast tissue for safety, and is usually followed by radiation treatment. Sometimes a surgeon can do a skin-sparing mastectomy, which makes
for a more natural appearance after reconstruction with an implant.
Some women have a *partial mastectomy*, a procedure that falls
somewhere in between the other two. In some cases, a woman may

have surgery for other reasons, or she may have abnormally formed breasts—these too, fall under the category of "reconstruction," but the surgery is usually less drastic, and what applies to the women who undergo mastectomies may not apply.

In most cases, lumpectomy is now considered to be as effective a treatment as mastectomy, particularly in women with early-stage breast cancer. However, there are still many cases in which a woman or her doctor opts for a mastectomy. More and more women who have mastectomies are electing to have breast reconstruction (approximately 114,000 in 2000), using an implant or their own body tissue to replace the lost breast or breasts. You can have breast reconstruction at any time after a mastectomy—one, five, ten, twenty, or more years later. A growing trend is to have immediate reconstruction while still under anesthesia from the cancer surgery. Another recent trend is for women at high risk for breast cancer to have prophylactic mastectomies and replace healthy breasts with implants. Some women have an implant inserted after a lumpectomy because even though their breast was "spared," their particular surgery removed so much tissue that their breasts appear abnormal.

Under the 1992 FDA ruling, implants of all types remained available to women who want reconstruction after surgery for breast cancer or other disease. Also included in this group are women with other medically defined deformities, such as those that cause asymmetry (one breast significantly smaller than the other) or those caused by an accident. The FDA also made silicone-gel implants available to women who previously had implants (either silicone-gel or saline) who wanted to replace them. While some women focus just on the life-and-death issues of breast cancer, others feel that breast cancer and mastectomy have been a major insult to them as a person. They may feel devastated by their situation, undesirable sexually, less confident, and ill at ease in sportswear and bathing suits. One woman told me about going to a nude beach: "The other women were either nude or topless. I went bottomless, but kept my top on. It was ridiculous!"

The ASPRS survey found that women who had their breasts reconstructed after cancer surgery listed three desires as their primary reasons for choosing implants:

♦ to free them from the need to wear an external prosthesis (90 percent)

♦ to help them forget about the state of their health (79 percent)

♦ to help them feel "whole" again (75 percent)

The survey found most of these expectations were met; 90 percent of the respondents agreed that they were indeed freed from the discomfort and inconvenience of an external prosthesis, and 80 percent said implants restored a feeling of "wholeness." However, while 55 percent said reconstruction also helped them forget that they had been diagnosed with cancer, this was significantly less than the 79 percent who had hoped for this benefit. In addition, a National Cancer Institute study published in 2000 found that reconstructive surgery was of less benefit to body image and psychological recovery than conventional wisdom would have us believe. The study involved detailed surveys of nearly two thousand breast cancer survivors. Women who had mastectomy-plus-reconstruction scored closer to the mastectomy-alone women than to the women who had breast-sparing lumpectomies. Women in the lumpectomy group reported fewer problems with their body image and feelings of sexual attractiveness than women in either mastectomy group. In fact, in some respects women with reconstruction fared worse than women without it—the negative sexual impact was 45 percent versus 30 percent for lumpectomy and 41 percent for mastectomy alone.

Here is how some women who lost a breast to cancer feel about reconstruction:

♦ The idea of reconstruction psychologically allowed me to have a mastectomy. There was never any question that I would have an implant, but no research about the implant was offered me. I remember waiting for my diagnosis in the doctor's office, striking up a conversation with an elegantly dressed older woman. She was having her second reconstruction. Would she show me? She would. She looked great in her bra and slip, but when she took them off—I was taken aback by all the scarring. But her attitude was so positive and encouraging, and that made me more upbeat. Because she had two reconstructions, what I failed to understand was what a single reconstructed breast would look like side by side with a healthy breast. I didn't realize that it would be a "wooden leg."

❖　When I was first diagnosed, I was upset by the idea of losing a breast, but I was much more upset by the idea of cancer taking my life. My breasts were not that important to me. I thought, if I have to lose any part of my body, an eye, a hand, a leg…these all seemed much worse than losing a breast, which, after all, served no practical function in most circumstances and was easily disguised by clothing. But later on it bothered me to be so lopsided. It felt odd and looked odd. When I got a good prosthesis, things looked up. But I still felt like a freak. When I heard about reconstruction, I knew that was for me….It would make me feel normal and whole again.

Women don't have to be big-breasted or particularly proud of, attached to, or focused on their breasts to feel the overwhelming loss. Norma Webb, an oncology nurse, writes in a 1994 article in *Innovations in Oncology Nursing* that she had assumed that since she had always been very small-breasted, the fact that she didn't have much to lose would allow her to adjust better to mastectomy than if she were a larger size. "I was certainly wrong about that!" she writes. "It is a great shock to look down and realize that a very visible part of you is gone, even if it is a small part."

Another breast cancer patient observed that after her reconstruction with saline implants, she now has a "maintenance-free chest and can utilize my energies in other ways."

In 1993, Eric Winer and his colleagues conducted a survey of 174 women who underwent breast reconstruction with silicone-gel implants. The women were selected at random and interviewed by telephone; all were aware of the controversy surrounding silicone implants. The researchers found that 76 percent felt reconstruction helped them cope better with breast cancer, but 57 percent were worried about the health effects. Only 16 percent had any regrets about the reconstruction; although 27 percent said they would choose silicone implants again, only 13 percent were considering having their implants removed.

While my prosthesis was better than nothing, every time I looked down at my chest, or put on my bra with the prosthesis, my stomach would lurch. I would be reminded I had cancer. Every time I took off my bra and the prosthesis, it was like having a mastectomy all over again. Having an implant changed all that. It's not perfect, but for me it's certainly much better than no breast. As is so often the case, there was one defining moment that made me certain that I did not want to live my life worrying about the state of my prosthesis. That moment came when I was body surfing in the Atlantic. I caught a really good wave and had an exhilarating ride, but the water was so turbulent that the force of it flipped over my prosthesis. The flat back of it was facing out! I submerged my body and managed to turn the form right side out again, but I wondered what I would have done if it had fallen out. Three hundred dollars tumbling around in the ocean. Would I have searched for it? Would I have asked for help? I didn't know, and I certainly did not look forward to more surgery, but I didn't want to repeat the incident.

## Breast Implants as Cosmetic Surgery: Augmentation

For better or worse, we live in a society that puts great emphasis on appearance. Numerous studies have shown that people prefer other people who meet a certain standard of attractiveness. This preference apparently knows no age boundaries. Judith Langlois, a psychologist at the University of Texas in Austin, found that the cuter the newborn infant, the more time the mother spent playing with the infant. She also found that infants will turn away from pictures of plain women and stare longer at pretty ones. When a similar experiment was repeated using a person with and without an ugly mask, Langlois got similar results. The pressure to fit into society's standards of beauty seems to begin in the cradle, if not sooner.

Throughout history, the breast has been equated with sexuality, femininity, womanliness, and the ability to nurture. Women's breasts have almost always played some role in what is perceived as being attractive. However, body "styles" go in and out of fashion, particularly in Western industrialized societies, and the size and shape of "ideal" breasts and their proportion with the rest of the body have shown considerable variation. A hundred years ago, plump was in. In the 1920s, the flapper look—smaller bust in relation to hips—was all the rage. In 1970, the "model" woman became taller and thinner.

At this moment in history, we mostly demand slim hips and large breasts. Although such a physique is very rare in nature, this image fairly screams at us day and night—on TV, at the movies, in magazines and newspapers, at the health club. Women: Buy this product and you will belong to the club of the attractive and slim-yet-well-endowed. Men: Buy this product and the well-endowed will flock to you.

Although breasts are undeniably the major sex symbol in our culture, plastic surgeons generally find that most women are not in search of the perfect "Playboy centerfold" body. The decision to have breast augmentation generally has nothing to do with making a sexual relationship better, and often the men in women's lives say, "I like you just the way you are—please don't do this for me."

Rather, both patients and their plastic surgeons feel that self-esteem and self-confidence are at the core of women's desire for breast augmentation. Fuller breasts often make women feel better about their bodies, more self-confident—and help them act more self-confident. Augmentation can be a self-fulfilling prophecy: When you project confidence, people react more positively to you.

Loren Eskenazi, a plastic surgeon in private practice in San Francisco, says:

> The vast majority of women who come in for either augmentation or reconstruction do so in spite of the views of their significant others. It's a red flag when a woman's significant other is pushing her or paying for it—you want to be careful about doing surgery for her because often such women will regret having done it. Women who choose to do this type of surgery for themselves usually are very determined to have it done. They rarely regret it.

Eskenazi says women who want breast surgery correlate what they see in the mirror with what they would like to feel like internally—"usually some combination of internal and external (societal) factors in terms of its drive. Nevertheless self-image is 100 percent real and needs to be valued."

When the ASPRS survey asked women why they chose to have breast augmentation, the three most common reasons given were:

◆ the desire for a more proportionate build (93 percent)

◆ a more appealing appearance (83 percent)

◆ a boost in self-confidence (76 percent)

The women felt that each of those expectations was met, with 95 percent of the respondents agreeing that their bodies looked more proportionate after surgery, 90 percent saying that they appeared more appealing, and 81 percent agreeing that they felt more confident.

The comments of women who had implants for cosmetic reasons illustrate these common themes:

> ◆   I never felt that I was too small; I originally went in for a breast lift. I'm a runner and my breasts had dropped at a very young age. I guess I just have that kind of breast tissue. My plastic surgeon told me that implants would lift me a little, too. He didn't push implants, he just showed me before and after photos and I noticed a significant difference in the

look—better cleavage, more roundness. So I decided to have implants.

◆   I had always been very, very flat-chested and I hated it. I always felt conscious, especially in high school. Why couldn't I just have enough to fill a bra? I was especially embarrassed in a bathing suit—the tops never fit me, so I'd wear the bottoms with a tube top. I found out my mother-in-law had implants, and I was amazed; I always thought they were real. I asked if I could touch them; they looked so real and felt so soft. I wanted implants too.

◆   I love them. I love the fact that I have breasts now. I don't think of them as implants; they're a part of me now. I'm just an average size, 34B, but I feel more than normal—I feel great! I feel so much better about myself. Sometimes I look at myself in the mirror and I say, "Oh! They're so lovely!" They're the breasts I would have been born with, if only they'd just grown a little.

The ASPRS survey, with its high level of reported satisfaction, took place before the implant controversy erupted. Neal Handel, a plastic surgeon formerly with the Breast Center in Van Nuys, California, wanted to find out how women felt about the possible health risks of implants in the new environment of heightened media attention and patient awareness. The results of his survey of eighty-five women who had breast augmentation were published in 1993. He and his fellow researchers came up with different figures from those of the ASPRS, but they still indicated that the majority of women were satisfied.

Handel found that most of the women's concerns related to doubts about the accuracy of mammography in an implanted breast, the possibility of leakage, and the question of arthritis or other autoimmune disorders. Specifically, 76 percent of women were either very concerned or somewhat concerned about implant safety, and only 2.4 percent were reassured by the media reports. The survey found only slight differences in women's feelings before and after hearing the negative media reports:

| Before the controversy | During the controversy |
|---|---|
| satisfied or very satisfied — 66% | satisfied or very satisfied — 61% |
| somewhat unsatisfied or very unsatisfied — 23% | somewhat unsatisfied or very unsatisfied — 32% |
| regretted having breast implants — 5% | regretted having breast implants — 9% |
| wanted their implants removed — 1% | wanted their implants removed — 6% |

The results of both of these surveys are remarkable, considering the rate of complications and repeat surgeries (see Chapters 4 and 5 for some of these statistics). Dr. Handel has not repeated his survey, but he says that after twenty-five years of experience he has observed that "The overwhelming majority are happy with their implants," and estimates that the percentage of those satisfied today is probably higher than 66 percent, because they are getting better results aesthetically. He continues, "A lot of people are willing to put up with the maintenance, the inconvenience, the possible need for additional surgery, the reality that they won't last forever, in exchange for the enhanced self-esteem and confidence." And the desire for beautiful breasts knows no age barrier, according to his story about one of his patients: "I had a 67-year-old unmarried patient who has had implants since 1975. Over the years, she has had a couple of deflations and replacements and finally had them removed altogether. She came back to me and said, 'I can't live like this. I just don't like the way I look.' Even though she has had three operations, she was willing to have a fourth to have them replaced."

## What the Breast-Implant Manufacturers Found

After the 1992 FDA ruling, the two major breast-implant manufacturers, Mentor and McGhan, conducted studies to determine the rate of complications (see Chapters 4 and 5) and the overall satisfaction and comfort with appearance, body image, self-esteem, and self-concept.

The McGhan studies found that:

◆ After eighteen months, out of the original 901 augmentation patients, 858 (95 percent) still had implants. After three years, 689 (76 percent) still had implants. Of these 689 patients, 655 (95 percent) indicated being satisfied with their breast-implant surgery. In other words, 24 percent (that's one out of four women) had them removed, presumably because of dissatisfaction or problems, or both;

◆ Before implantation, the 689 patients scored higher (better) than the general U.S. female population on SF-36 and MOS-20, tests that measure general health-related quality of life. But three years after augmentation, their scores were worse. According to two other tests, the Tennessee Self-Concept Scale (which measures overall self-concept) and the Body Esteem Scale (which measures overall self-esteem related specifically to one's body), the women showed no changes over the three years. According to two more tests, the Rosenberg Self-Esteem Scale (which measures overall self-esteem) and the Semantic Differential Scale (which measures attitudes about one's breasts compared to attitudes about oneself), the women showed only a slight increase. In other words, they scored worse after implants or did not feel significantly better about themselves after implants, exploding the widely held conception that implants enhance self-image and confidence;

◆ For reconstruction patients, 169 out of the original 237 patients (71 percent) still had implants and were in the study after three years. Of these 169 patients, 149 (88 percent) indicated that they were satisfied with their breast-implant surgery. In other words, 29 percent (one out of three) of the women had their implants removed, presumably because they had problems or were dissatisfied with the results. And among those who kept them, 12 percent (one out of ten) were dissatisfied.

The Mentor study tested women before and three years after surgery. It found:

◆ After three years, out of the original 1,264 augmentation patients, 955 (76 percent) still had implants. Of the 955 patients still in the study, 860 (90 percent) indicated being satisfied with the general appearance of their breasts, as measured by the Breast Evaluation Questionnaire (BEQ). In other words, 24 percent (one out of four women) had them removed, presumably because they were dissatisfied, or had problems, or both; and of those who kept their implants, one out of ten was dissatisfied;

◆ Most augmentation patients who still had their original implants and were still in the study at three years exhibited an improvement in the two measured subscales of the Multidimensional Body–Self Relation Questionnaire (MBSRQ; which measures comfort with one's general appearance). For augmentation patients, the Tennessee Self-Concept Scale showed only a slight increase at three years compared to before implantation;

◆ For reconstruction patients, out of the original 416 patients, 283 (68 percent) still had implants and were in the study after three years, while 32 percent (one out of three women) had their implants removed, presumably because they were dissatisfied, had problems, or both.

While these percentages are nothing to write home about to begin with, we must also remember that they relate only to the women who still had implants. In both studies, after three years, about 30 percent of the women who had reconstruction and about 24 percent of the women who had augmentation no longer had their implants—presumably because of complications or because they were unhappy with the results. They show that a large percentage of women keep their implants even though they are not satisfied with them. And note that the McGhan studies show that an additional 19 percent of participants had their implants removed between eighteen months and three years after implantation—a significant, perhaps even dramatic, difference.

## So Where Are We Now?

As of this writing, the FDA has formally approved the use of saline-filled implants made by two companies, Mentor and McGhan, in all women for either augmentation or reconstruction purposes. All other manufacturers' saline-filled implants are considered to be investigational or experimental. Silicone-gel implants are available for women seeking breast reconstruction or revision of an existing breast implant—either silicone-gel- or saline-filled. Therefore, women who can have gel-filled implants include women who have had breast cancer surgery (partial or modified mastectomy or lumpectomy), a severe injury to the breast, a birth defect that affects the breast, or a medical condition causing a severe breast abnormality. Also, women who wish to have a breast implant replaced for a medical reason (such as a rupture) may also get silicone-gel implants. In addition, a few thousand women are eligible to get silicone-gel implants for first-time augmentation.

# 3

# Types of Breast Implants and Surgical Procedures

There are two basic types of implants used today: silicone-gel-filled and saline-filled. Most of the implants used today are filled with saline—since 1993 about 90 to 95 percent of them. Before that, 90 to 95 percent of implants were silicone gel. Today, silicone-gel-filled implants are available only under certain circumstances, but many women already have them, or are considering getting them. In this chapter, you'll learn the basics about these two main types of implants and a few variations. You'll also learn about the different types of surgeries used to insert the implants in the body, both for augmentation (breast enlargement) and reconstruction (re-creation of a breast after it has been surgically removed).

## Types of Implants

In both saline-filled and silicone-gel-filled implants, the filling is contained within envelopes or sacs made of a soft rubbery form of silicone called an *elastomer*.

## Silicone-Gel-Filled Implants

These implants consist of an elastomer envelope prefilled (before surgery) with a clear, sticky, thick jellylike form of silicone that closely approximates the consistency of breast tissue. Before the 1992 FDA ruling, this was the most common type of implant. Silicone-gel implants come in many sizes; the size used depends on the amount of augmentation desired or the size the reconstructed breast is to be. Much of the controversy surrounding implants is related to the possible adverse effects when the silicone gel leaks, bleeds, or ruptures through the elastomer envelope.

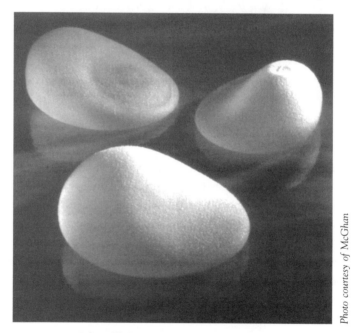

*Photo courtesy of McGhan*

*Saline-filled implants, with textured shells*

## Saline-Filled Implants

These implants contain saline, a sterile salt water. The implant is surgically inserted while empty and is filled after it is put in place, which allows for some adjustment in size. According to some, the major drawback of saline implants is that they do not feel or look as natural as gel implants. This is especially true in women who have little tissue left to cover the implant after a mastectomy. Some women say the implant tends to wrinkle or ripple under the skin, and that the breast doesn't move or hang naturally—it sloshes. In addition, many of the older saline implants had a higher rate of leaking and deflation than silicone-gel implants, which means more frequent surgery to replace them. On the other hand, most surgeons believe that if the saline does leak into the body, it is similar to other body fluids and is likely to be absorbed without harm. It is now well established that saline implants do not always stay sterile throughout the life of the implants, and this might also pose health risks, but of a different nature than the silicone gel, as you will see in Chapter 5.

Not everyone has found that saline implants of any age are more prone to either wrinkling or leaking than are silicone implants. Among these is Paul Striker, a New York plastic surgeon who has used saline implants almost exclusively for more than thirty years. According to Striker, saline's main disadvantage is a psychological one—if the implant ruptures, it deflates immediately and sometimes completely, which can be unacceptable to some women. "Others couldn't care less and feel it's a good trade-off for the added safety of saline," he says. He also likes the fact that a smaller incision is needed to insert the implant.

## Double-Lumen Implants

These implants consist of two lumens—or envelopes—one inside the other. In some models, the inner envelope is prefilled with silicone gel, and the outer envelope is filled with saline at the time of surgery. In other models, the relationship is reversed and the inner envelope is filled with saline. Some studies suggest that the double-walled model results in a softer, more natural appearance because it reduces the incidence of capsular contracture (see Chapter 4). A small number of triple-lumen implants (with two inner layers of silicone gel) were used at one time. I had a double-lumen implant originally in 1982, but double lumens are no longer available in the United States.

## Polyurethane Foam–Coated Implants

According to the FDA, about 110,000 women have or had implants covered with polyurethane foam. This was meant to be an improvement over the standard silicone implant, which has a smooth outer surface. The foam was thought to reduce incidence of capsular contracture because the texture encouraged the body tissue to grow into it. However, the foam, which was identical to that used in furniture upholstery, oil filters, and carburetors, was found to increase risk of infection, fragment in the body, and chemically break down and release small amounts of a substance called 2-toluenediamine (TDA). TDA is known to cause cancer in animals and was removed from hair dyes many years ago. These implants are no longer available. One study found that a woman's risk of cancer from exposure to TDA released by an implant would be about one in a million over the course of her lifetime; however, others, including scientists at the FDA, thought the risk was much higher than that.

## Textured Implants

Many of today's implants have textured silicone surfaces, which are also thought to reduce capsular contracture. Since no foam is involved, they do not pose the potential risks of the foam-coated models.

## Soy-Oil-Filled Implants

In the mid-nineties, a new type of implant was introduced that was less radiopaque (that is, it didn't block the X-ray beam of a mammography as thoroughly; see Chapter 4) and made of a "natural" substance—soybean oil. Dr. Neal Handel was one of the five U.S. investigators who in 1994 and 1995 implanted eleven out of the total of fifty women who participated in the study. In addition, over five thousand European women were implanted. Dr. Handel says, "The mammograms were great—you could see right through the filler. The cosmetic result was okay—a bit firm, some wrinkling. Overall, the patient satisfaction was high." But they soon proved to be a disaster. In early 2000 there were reports that rancid soy oil was leaking out of the implants, and all women were advised to remove them as quickly as possible. In two of the four women from whom he's removed the implants thus far, Dr. Handel recalls, "There was gross leakage of the material outside the implant, and it created material that was like cream cheese—fatty, granular, yellowish." He says it was never proven to be toxic, but the hypothetical concern made the FDA and the Medical Devices Agency (the British equivalent of the FDA) ban the implants. Soybean-oil implants—called "tofu titties" in England—have gone the way of the Edsel.

## Implant Surgery

Surgery for implantation varies as to the location of the incision and the location of the implants (above or beneath the pectoralis muscle). Women undergoing reconstruction have additional options as well; for them, other types of breast surgeries may be done to improve the overall effect. These additional options and surgeries are covered later in this chapter, in the section titled "Related Techniques and Surgeries for Reconstruction."

### Simple Implantation

Implant surgery for breast augmentation involves making a single incision in or near the breast and inserting the implant either between the breast and the chest muscle (pectoralis major) or behind the muscle. This is also the simplest type of surgery that is used for breast reconstruction; in this case, the implant is most often placed behind the muscle. When used for reconstruction, it works best in women whose opposite breast is of small or medium size and not very pendulous.

### Incision Locations

The location of the incision depends on the type of surgery (reconstruction or augmentation), your body type, and your personal preference. The most commonly used incision for augmentation is in the crease under the breast because the scar is easily hidden and is closest to the blood supply. However, the scar left by this type of incision tends to be wide and sometimes dark in color, although it may fade with time. An incision may be made around the areola; such an incision tends to result in a thinner, lighter scar that

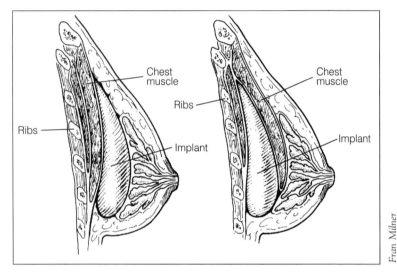

*Breast implants are placed either between the breast and the chest muscle or behind the chest muscle.*

is concealed by the color of the areola, but when this scar heals poorly, it is quite visible. The third possibility, an incision under the arm, leaves the breast completely unscarred, but it creates a scar under the arm, which may be prominent. This approach is also more difficult surgically and may lead to bleeding, improper placement of the implant, or other complications.

Women who have had a mastectomy can usually avoid receiving another incision and scar because the surgeon can make the reconstruction incision along part of the mastectomy scar.

## The Surgery

Surgery may be done under either local or general anesthesia, in the hospital, in a surgical center, or in the physician's office. It is usually done as one-day outpatient surgery; however, for some

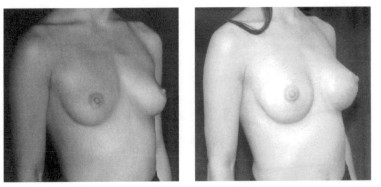

*Photos courtesy of Loren Eskenazi, M.D.*

*Before and after breast augmentation with implants*

women an overnight stay is recommended. The procedure takes two hours or more, depending on whether the implant goes above or beneath the muscle. The surgeon creates a pocket—a space between the tissues—to accommodate the implant. After inserting the implant, he or she closes the pocket and sutures the tissues in place. Then either a surgical bra or a bandage is placed over the incision. Postsurgical swelling is to be expected, as is some pain and discomfort. The degree varies from person to person and can sometimes be quite severe. Most women return to work and resume nonstrenuous activities, such as driving, about a week to ten days after surgery.

My reconstruction involved this simple type of surgery, since my breasts were not particularly large and I had enough skin and muscle elasticity after the mastectomy to accommodate an implant. As with any surgery, experiences vary greatly—I have heard of women who bounced right back and did laundry the day after this simple surgery, and of others who were bedridden for days afterward. I was very "up" for this surgery, in contrast to my feelings about the surgery to remove my breast. However, when I awoke from the anesthesia, I could not believe the intense pain in my chest. It felt as though the creature in the movie *Alien* was trying to burst out. No one told me there would be so much pain, and I was very angry at the time. Much to my surprise and relief, the pain vanished in an hour or two, and I required little or no pain

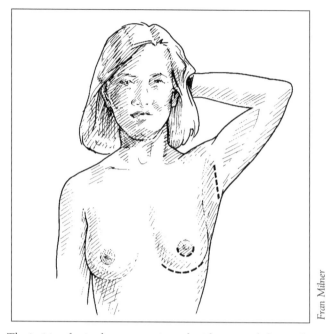

*Fran Milner*

*The incision for implant surgery is made either around the areola, along the breast fold, or under the arm; for reconstruction, a fourth option is to make the incision along the mastectomy scar.*

medication after that initial episode. I went home that night, and the next day I was up and about.

## Related Techniques and Surgeries for Reconstruction

Most natural breasts have varying degrees of pendulousness, or droop (*ptosis* in medicalese); where the breast meets the chest, there is a crease (*inframammary fold*). Many women undergoing reconstruction do not have enough tissue remaining after mastectomy to allow an implant to be successfully inserted using the relatively simple procedure described above. Simple implantation results in a relatively small breast that sits high on the chest. Instead of the natural pendulousness, the reconstructed breast is suspiciously perky, even when the surgery is otherwise "successful." The mastectomy may have removed a lot of skin and muscle, or the skin may not be naturally elastic, or radiation therapy may have changed the elasticity. The opposite breast may be too large to match the reconstructed breast, or it may have much more droop.

Several techniques have been designed to deal with the problem of too little tissue at the mastectomy site. Procedures also exist to help women obtain a better match with the unaffected breast and to create a new nipple on the reconstructed breast. Some procedures involve the transfer of tissue from the back, belly, or buttocks and often do not require using an implant at all.

## Tissue Expansion

This common variation of the simple surgical implantation uses a special type of implant called a *tissue expander*. Like an implant, a tissue expander has a rubber silicone outer shell. It is surgically inserted into the pocket, often through a small incision in the mastectomy scar. Over the course of several months, the surgeon adds small amounts of saline through a special tube. This gradually inflates the expander like a balloon, gently expanding the skin and muscle by stimulating the growth of healthy new tissue. This procedure creates a more natural appearance and may reduce the risk of capsular contracture (hardening of the breast). Many women say they feel some pressure or discomfort after each expansion

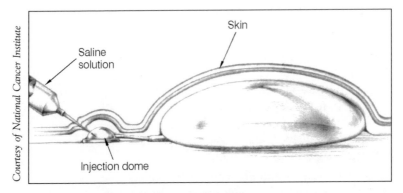

*Tissue expander being filled after implantation*

session, and some feel a great deal of pain, but this diminishes as the tissue expands to accommodate the added saline.

Tissue expanders may be temporary or permanent. When sufficient tissue has been created, the temporary expander is surgically removed and a more permanent implant is inserted. This requires a second surgery, which is usually done under general anesthesia but may also be done under local anesthesia on an outpatient basis. There is also a more permanent version of the tissue expander. It consists of an outer shell of silicone gel and an inner shell that is gradually filled with saline after implantation. It is designed with a special filling device that is removed under local anesthesia after inflation is complete, which causes an internal valve to close automatically. The permanent expander thus avoids a second surgery.

The downside of tissue expansion is that the expander is usually overfilled about 200 milliliters larger than the opposite breast in order to achieve a more natural droop. It is kept overfilled for six weeks to several months to allow the tissues to fully adjust, and some women are embarrassed during this time by the discrepancy in size with the opposite breast. And, as we shall see later in this chapter, even with an expanded pocket to receive an implant, the results are often disappointing or lead to complications, such as capsular contracture.

This thirty-four-year-old woman describes what it was like for her to undergo immediate reconstruction with a tissue expander:

> When I woke from the surgery, it felt like I had a hot-water bottle under my skin. There was an adolescent mound, no nipple, but at least there was the beginning of a process, a growth that would unfold. I wore the expander for about five months. It felt like I was wearing a long-line bra—not painful, but uncomfortable. As the day of my permanent implant approached, I grew nervous. Because I knew that when I woke up from that, whatever I had would be "it"— what I would have to live with, not something temporary anymore. It was just a continuation of the weirdness of it all.

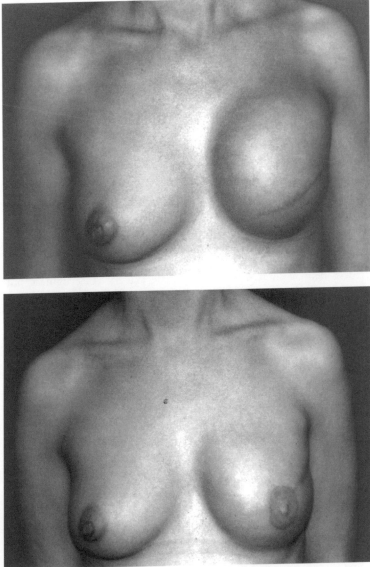

*Breast reconstruction with an implant.*
**Top:** *The patient is temporarily overexpanded to develop a pocket for the implant.* **Bottom:** *Finished reconstruction, including a nipple and areola.*

I resented having to massage it, that it required continual effort on my part. That I couldn't really forget it. But this gradually helped me integrate the implant into my life and my body.

## Tissue-Flap Surgeries

A burgeoning category of breast surgery involves the transferring of tissue from another part of the body. Using these techniques, surgeons can transfer a flap of skin, muscle, blood vessels, and fat from the upper back, abdomen, or buttocks either to create a larger, sturdier pocket for an implant or to fashion the entire breast and thus avoid using an implant altogether. These more complicated flap techniques are growing more popular—not only to create breasts with a more natural shape and feel, but to allow reconstruction in women who have so little skin or such tight, irradiated skin that reconstruction would otherwise be impossible or unsatisfactory. Tissue-flap techniques are also offered to women who don't want to worry about the adverse effects of implants, who may be at higher risk for silicone sensitivity, or who have already suffered adverse implant effects but do not want to give up reconstruction entirely.

Using tissue from your own body (*autogenous* tissue) may seem an ideal solution. But as with everything there are trade-offs: These procedures are major operations that are more extensive than a mastectomy. They are generally much more complicated, more expensive, and more risky than a simple implantation even with an expander. They require longer hospital stays and recuperative time. They also leave you with more scars on your breasts and on the donor site from where the flap was taken, and the results are variable. Nevertheless, they offer a third reconstruction option— in addition to simple implantation and tissue expansion—that more and more women are choosing. These surgeries should be considered only if you are in good general health, are strongly motivated, are not very overweight or underweight, do not smoke, and have good circulation.

Incredibly, the flap technique was developed as long ago as 1906, by an Italian, sixteen years after the first radical mastectomy was performed. We have come a long way since then. But even surgeons who are avid promoters of these procedures are quick to point out that there is a learning curve with them. The techniques are evolving and the results are getting better while the risk of complications is lessening. Although some surgeons are horrified at the extensiveness of the surgery, others feel the results are worth the risk—in the right patient. In the past, most of these procedures were reserved for women for whom a simple implantation was impossible or extremely risky, or who had previously endured problems with implants. Today, they are being offered for a broader range of circumstances, including immediate reconstruction. When performed by a capable surgeon, these procedures have made some women very happy.

The two most common types of flap surgery performed today are the TRAM flap, in which tissue is taken from the abdomen, and the latissimus dorsi flap, which takes tissue from the upper back. The latissimus procedure is the simpler of the two and formerly was the most popular. But because it usually still requires using an implant, it has been superceded by the TRAM, which usually does not require an implant.

## Latissimus Dorsi (Back Muscle) Flap

This procedure was very common before tissue expansion became popular and still may be used when more tissue is needed than an expander can create. The surgery involves transferring skin, muscle, fat, and the blood vessels that nourish them from the back to the breast area. The surgeon surgically creates a "flap" of skin, fat, and the latissimus dorsi muscle (the broad, flat, triangular-shaped back muscle that moves the arm, draws the shoulder back and down, and helps draw the body up when climbing). The flap is then "tunneled" inside the body from the back to the front of the chest. The skin and muscle remain partly attached to the blood and nerve supply. The tissue flap is set into the mastectomy site and is sutured in place. Originally, this procedure was used to

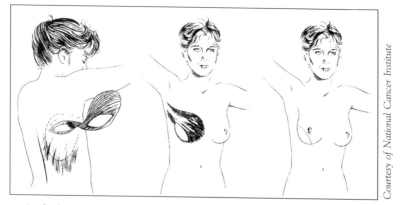

Courtesy of National Cancer Institute

*In the latissimus dorsi flap procedure, the surgeon removes skin, fat, and muscle from the back and transfers them to the breast area.*

create a pocket for an implant. The extra tissue generally allows a larger implant to be inserted and creates a softer breast with a more natural shape. New techniques may take enough fat from the back to form a breast mound and avoid using an implant.

This procedure is done in the hospital under general anesthesia. It creates an incision on the back, which heals to a pencil-thin scar that is covered by most clothing. The procedure takes about two to four hours and requires a hospital stay of five to six days. There is usually considerably more discomfort than after a simple implantation, and patients take longer to recuperate—five to six weeks. There is a risk (about 2 percent) that the blood vessels feeding the flap could become blocked or twisted and that the transferred tissue could die. In addition, the procedure may weaken the back and shoulder muscles, and a nerve may be injured during surgery, which may cause "shoulder droop."

A study by Frankie Fraulin and colleagues tested both men and women who had surgery involving the transfer of the latissimus dorsi muscle. Their thirty subjects used special machines that tested the affected shoulder under various conditions and simulated four activities that involve latissimus dorsi function: ladder climbing, painting overhead, pushing up from a chair, and cross-country skiing. They found that these "dynamic muscle tests demonstrate a deficit of muscle power and endurance" following

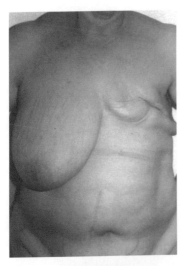

*Reconstruction with an extended latissimus dorsi flap.*
**Top:** *After a modified radical mastectomy.* **Center:** *After reconstruction, which did not include an implant, but did include a breast lift on the right side (mastopexy).*
**Bottom:** *The back view, showing the scar at the donor site.*

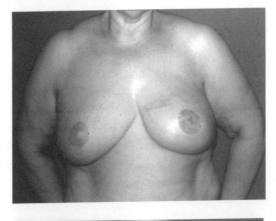

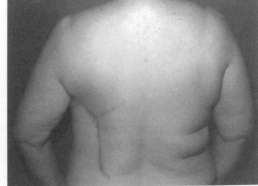

*Photos courtesy of Stephen S. Kroll, M.D.*

transfer of the muscle. In addition, some patients complain that the muscle transfer leaves their back feeling tight on the affected side. It appears that women who are very active physically—particularly in sports requiring upper-body strength such as golf, swimming, and tennis—will miss their latissimus dorsi, especially if the surgery is on their dominant side.

A variation of the standard latissimus dorsi flap procedure, developed by Edward W. Knowlton, chief of plastic surgery at John Muir Hospital, is called the PEG procedure. It requires that the general surgeon do a skin-sparing mastectomy and cut the skin only around the outer border of the areola. When done as an immediate reconstruction, this one-step procedure results in a scar on the back but none on the breast except for the incision around the areola. When done as a delayed reconstruction, it avoids creating an additional breast scar. In either case, Knowlton says, in the majority of patients there may be enough autologous tissue to reconstruct a breast without using an implant. He says he can also avoid operating on the healthy breast to achieve a closer match to the reconstructed breast (see "Surgery to Improve Symmetry," later in this chapter) and argues that other muscles easily compensate for the absence of the muscle in the back.

## TRAM Flap (Abdominal Muscle)

In this procedure, the surgeon creates a flap using skin, fat, and one or both of the rectus abdominis muscles, hence the name *transverse rectus abdominis muscle* (TRAM) *flap*. This pair of muscles extends the length of the front of the stomach and flexes the spinal column, tenses the stomach and intestine walls, and helps press the contents of the stomach and intestines. In the original (conventional) TRAM flap procedure, the flap remains attached to the original blood supply and is tunneled through the abdomen up to the breast area. In the newer free-flap procedure, the tissue is detached from the abdominal blood supply and reconnected to the blood vessels in the axilla (armpit) using microvascular surgery.

In some cases, the tissue is used to create a pocket that more comfortably accommodates an implant. But often this procedure is used because the abdomen contains enough fatty tissue to create a new breast mound and avoid using an implant altogether.

As with the back flap, the TRAM procedure is performed under general anesthesia. However, it is a much more extensive surgery that takes up to between eight and twelve hours to perform. Excessive bleeding may occur, and many women bank their own blood prior to the procedure as a precaution to avoid needing a transfusion. The TRAM procedure carries a higher risk of surgical complications, and requires a longer recovery period than other reconstruction surgeries. Generally, patients require a hospital stay of two to five days, then six to eight weeks of recovery

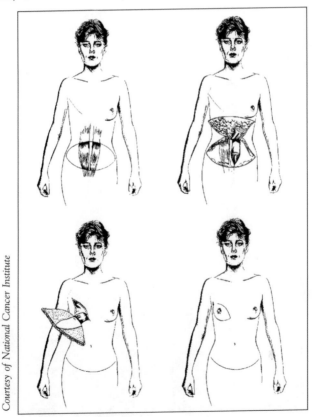

*Courtesy of National Cancer Institute*

*In the abdominal flap procedure, the surgeon removes skin, fat, and muscle from the abdomen and transfers them to the breast area.*

time at home, but some women find they need a full year to get back to normal activity. Some women are surprised by the intensity of the postsurgical pain, and most women require a good deal of pain medication. Some plastic surgeons tell patients they get a bonus with the procedure, a "tummy tuck." But the result is not really the same as a true tummy tuck, and it leaves a long scar across the abdomen from one hip to the other. In addition, it may weaken the abdominal wall and so cause a hernia. To avoid this, a plastic mesh may be installed where the muscle was removed. The patient may be unable to stand up straight right away after surgery. The surgery may also cause a temporary or permanent loss of abdominal muscle strength. And it may be inappropriate for patients who plan to become pregnant in the future.

In the TRAM flap's early days, surgeons believed the procedure was unsuitable for women who were very slim, who had undergone previous abdominal surgery, who had diabetes, or who smoked heavily. Today, many feel the only women who do not qualify are women with uncontrolled cancer, who are extremely obese, or who have other severe medical problems that make elective surgery too risky. Even diabetes, with its attendant blood-circulation and

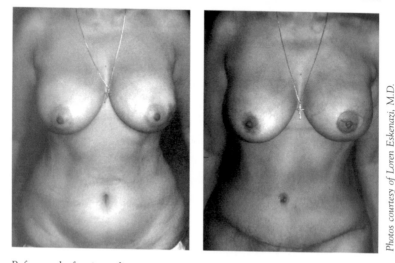

*Photos courtesy of Loren Eskenazi, M.D.*

*Before and after immediate reconstruction of the left breast with a conventional TRAM flap (the before photo shows bruising from a biopsy)*

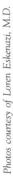

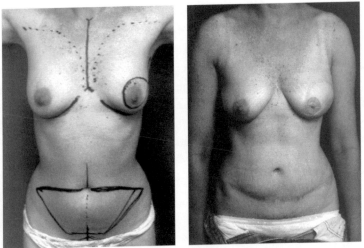

*Before and after immediate right breast reconstruction with a free TRAM flap. Since the surgeon is highly skilled in this technique, the reconstructed breast resembles the naural breast very closely*

healing problems, may no longer prevent a woman from having a TRAM, particularly the free-flap version, according to some surgeons. Smokers, however, are asked to abstain for a few weeks before and after the surgery to decrease the risk of necrosis (death) of the flap tissue.

There is some evidence that immediate reconstruction and the free-flap technique may increase the success of the TRAM flap procedure. L. Franklyn Elliot led a team that performed a series of immediate breast reconstructions using the TRAM flap. Patients received either free-flap or conventional TRAMs. Of the free-flap group, the women experienced shorter hospitalization times, fewer infections, and fewer abdominal hernias; and fewer women lost the transplanted fat tissue than in the conventional group. Based on the results of this study and of other studies, researchers believe the free-flap procedure is particularly successful for immediate reconstruction. There is more blood flow to the free flap, and the blood vessels are easier to find and use since they are not imbedded in scar tissue.

A simpler way to add skin and fat to the lower portion of the breast is to use tissue from an area of the midriff just below the breast. This older approach leaves a visible scar along the midriff and so would not appeal to women who expose this area, for example, by wearing two-piece bathing suits. However, this type of flap offers several advantages over the other two, newer, more popular flap techniques. It avoids using any muscle, eliminates the need for tissue expanders, and the color of the skin is a better match.

## Gluteal Free Flap

A third type of flap procedure—by far the least commonly used flap technique—involves transferring tissue from the upper buttock area to the breast area. Either the upper or lower half of the gluteus maximus muscle, along with the overlying fat and skin, is transferred as a free flap, with no tunneling. When the upper muscle is used, it leaves a noticeable scar and indentation in the buttock. When the lower portion is used, it leaves a flattened buttock, noticeably different from the opposite buttock in tight clothing such as bathing suits and pants. It also is more complicated and expensive and has a higher failure rate than the TRAM procedure, and is therefore only attempted when other techniques are inappropriate, either because the patient has had prior abdominal surgery or because she is too thin.

## Which Reconstruction Technique Is Best?

Few studies have compared the results of the various reconstruction techniques. A 1989 study by J. B. McCraw and colleagues asked patients to rate the results of their reconstructions. They reported a higher rate of complications and less satisfactory results after tissue expansion than after the TRAM flap. Another study by P. B. Rosen and colleagues, published in 1990, revealed similar complication rates between the two procedures, but the authors felt the aesthetic results were better with the TRAM flap. R. E. Mansel and colleagues published a study in 1986 in which the sur-

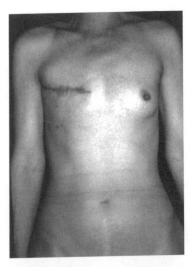

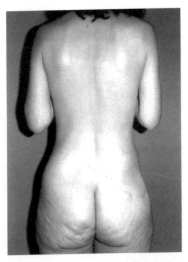

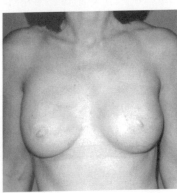

Reconstruction using a gluteal free flap. **Top left:** After a right modified radical mastectomy. **Top right:** The healed donor site after taking tissue from the upper right gluteal area. **Bottom:** The result of reconstruction of the right breast with the gluteal flap. (The left breast also had a subsequent mastectomy for a second cancer and immediate reconstruction with a saline implant.)

geons preferred the results after immediate reconstruction with TRAM flaps to those obtained using tissue expansion.

Another study, by Stephen S. Kroll and Bonnie Baldwin, published in 1992, evaluated 287 women (325 reconstructions) and the three techniques used most frequently at the University of Texas M. D. Anderson Cancer Center: tissue expansion with silicone implant (105 breasts), latissimus dorsi flap (47 breasts, including 5 without an implant), and the TRAM flap. All surgeries were performed by Dr. Kroll, and were graded on a scale from 1 to 4 (excellent to poor) using post-operative photographs. Individual criteria were symmetry, shape, ptosis (droop), and scarring; an over-all grade assessed the success of the procedure as a whole. Unlike previous studies, the judging was done by independent observers who were not members of the surgical team. Their results are summarized as follows:

The TRAM flaps received the best overall grade (2.07), the latissimus dorsi was second best (2.21), and the tissue expansion came in third (2.57). On an aesthetic scale, scarring was least in those with tissue expanders, but breast shape and droop were better with the flap procedures. Breasts appeared more symmetrical in patients who had immediate reconstruction because the surgeon was able to preserve breast tissue and knew where to place the inframammary fold. In this study, tissue expansion was used most often for immediate reconstruction, and this probably raised its success rate. If only immediate reconstruction had been considered, the authors state, the TRAM flap would have scored even higher. However, they also point out that most tissue-expansion failures occurred when using older smooth-walled devices, and that the failure rate might have been lower with textured implants.

The researchers found that each technique had its own advantages, risks, and complications. They write that although they were forced to compare "apples and oranges," such comparisons are desperately needed because otherwise surgeons cannot make fair recommendations to their patients. They point out that tissue expansion is probably the most widely used technique in North America because it is relatively simple, quick, convenient, and does not cause scars or loss of muscle function. Although in some women the results are as good as with autogenous tissue transfer, many patients develop capsular contracture and inadequate expansion; because an implant is required, there may also be late complications such as infection or the implant pushing through the skin (extrusion). In this study, 21 percent of the tissue expansions failed because of these complications, versus a 3 percent failure rate for the TRAM flap and 9 percent for the latissimus dorsi flap. At M. D. Anderson, surgeons have noticed that while the latissimus dorsi procedure has a relatively low rate of early complications, it has a "disturbingly high" rate of late capsular contracture and local infection.

The researchers admit that the TRAM flap is complex and expensive; it requires longer hospital stays and recovery time than the other two procedures; complications can be severe; and the technique is more demanding, particularly for the free-flap procedure. However, they feel their study suggests that "the additional costs and more extensive surgery are justified by the low failure rate, the aesthetic success of the outcomes, and a long-term freedom from late complications." For the average patient, the TRAM flap is "generally the method of choice."

These surgeons are using the latissimus dorsi less often than they once did (primarily they use it in obese women, or in those who want to avoid implants but for whom the TRAM flap would be too risky). In such cases, they favor the extended latissimus dorsi procedure, which does not require an implant. They generally prefer tissue expansion in women who are over sixty-five, for whom extensive surgery is too risky, and for those who do not want the extra scarring inherent in the flap procedures. They state that "the experience of reconstructive surgeons over many decades with foreign bodies of many varieties...suggests that no implants, however ingenious, are likely to be tolerated by the human body as well as autogenous tissue."

## Surgery to Improve Symmetry

Breast reconstruction leaves a simple mound that may not match the other breast in size or level. For some women, this is acceptable. Others prefer the reconstruction to look more like a breast and to match the remaining breast. This means additional surgeries to add an areola and a nipple and to lift and perhaps reduce the size of the other breast.

The surgeon may construct a nipple using skin and connective tissue from the chest, groin, earlobe, or the nipple of the opposite breast. Many women have the skin surrounding the new nipple dyed to resemble an areola, using a special tattooing technique.

All these procedures may be done in the surgeon's office under local anesthesia.

Even after a nipple is added, a reconstructed breast never matches the other breast exactly. Asymmetry is less of a problem when a woman has had a double mastectomy and two implants. But a woman with one natural breast and one synthetic breast may be bothered that they obviously do not feel or look the same. The reconstructed breast is generally rounder, higher, and firmer than the natural one. It may also be smaller because of the limited amount of tissue left to receive the implant. As a result, some women choose to have additional surgery to lift the natural breast to a higher position (mastopexy) or to reduce its size (reduction mastopexy) to achieve a breast that better matches the reconstructed one in size and shape.

Often, even if the result of the reconstruction is nearly symmetrical, the symmetry is fleeting. So even though a patient may not need a mastopexy at the time of reconstruction, as time goes by, she may want to consider this additional surgery on her healthy breast as gravity exerts its pull on the natural breast, but not the reconstructed one. As the authors of a study published in 2001 wrote, "[T]he long-term cosmetic outcome of breast implant reconstruction is unknown." They evaluated 344 women who had undergone immediate reconstruction. One of the results they found was that the overall cosmetic effect deteriorated steadily over the course of nine years. Initially 86 percent of the women had acceptable results at the two-year mark, but this had dwindled to only 54 percent at the five-year mark. One factor was capsular contracture, but even in women with no or little capsular contracture, their breasts looked more and more uneven with the passing years because their natural breast continued to get droopier, while the reconstructed breast stayed firm and high.

A surgeon may suggest using a tissue expander to increase symmetry and to minimize the need for a mastopexy, but this is usually only temporarily effective. The flap surgeries explained earlier are often able to achieve a closer match initially and, unlike a simple reconstruction, the symmetry may hold for the rest of the patient's life. This is why Melvin Spira, professor of surgery in the Division of Plastic Surgery at the Baylor College of Medicine, in Houston, Texas, is not alone when he says, "I prefer to use natural tissue for reconstruction if possible. It's almost impossible to get any lasting symmetry when you use an implant," because the tight skin can only stretch so much.

No matter which surgery you choose, be prepared for a recuperation time that may last longer than you expect. All of my breast cancer–related surgeries—mastectomy, initial implantation, mastopexy, nipple reconstruction, explantation of my silicone implant and replacement with saline—were more painful and took longer to heal than I had hoped or was led to believe. And I am a trooper and a good healer! Especially if you have breast reconstruction, I urge you to learn about the special exercises and movements that can help you retain and regain your strength and flexibility, and minimize tightness and pain. For more information about recovering from breast cancer surgeries, see *Recovering from Breast Surgery*, by Diana Stumm, PT. I also recommend *Lymphedema: A Breast Cancer Patient's Guide to Prevention and Healing* by Jeanne Burt and Gwen White, PT. This book helps breast cancer patients prevent and/or heal lymphedema, a disfiguring, painful swelling, most frequently of the arm, that affects approximately 25 percent of breast cancer surgery patients.

# 4

# Effects of Implants on Nearby Tissue (Local Complications)

Potential problems with breast implants fall into two broad categories: those that occur in tissue near the implants or in the implants themselves (local complications or symptoms), and those that affect the whole body (systemic disease, addressed in the next chapter). The local complications covered in this chapter include breast hardening (capsular contracture); leaking, rupture, and deflation; and infection. That these problems plague many women with implants is no longer contested—it is obvious that these occur much more frequently than previously thought and generally occur to some degree in most women with implants. Less accepted and harder to measure—and therefore more controversial—are the systemic problems. So, perhaps a better way of labeling these complications would be "known" and "unknown" or "confirmed" and "unconfirmed." Some experts feel that the problems should be thought of as existing on a continuum, with local complications preceding and leading to systemic disease.

However, even with regard to the better-acknowledged and less controversial local effects, there is uncertainty and disagreement. The reason the information is so sketchy is that no one has been keeping track of women with implants. Most of the data we have so far come from studies of small numbers of women, or animal studies that may or may not be applicable to humans, or anecdotal reports of individual cases. Another problem is that most women lose contact with their surgeons over time and so are not monitored for the length of time it would take for certain complications to show up. In addition, many women have been reluctant to report implant problems, or their physicians have not made the connection between women's implants and their health problems.

The Institute of Medicine report published in 1999 and mentioned in Chapter 1 stated that local complications were the primary safety issue with implants, and that these have not been well studied.

Unfortunately, the studies conducted thus far rarely study women with reconstruction separately from women with augmentation. However, in studies that do make an attempt to examine these women as two separate groups, women who have had implants for reconstruction appear to be at higher risk than women having implants for augmentation. Women having immediate reconstruction with a silicone implant fare worst of all, according to the Institute of Medicine report issued in 1999. The risk seems to be even greater in patients who have had tissue expanders, and probably also in those who have had radiation to the area.

Complications often mean additional surgery, either with or without replacement of the troublesome implant(s). In a study of both saline and silicone implants, on average 24 percent of women underwent additional surgery within the first five years after receiving their initial implants. In this study, one out of eight augmentation patients required the surgery, and one out of three reconstruction patients.

According to studies of saline implants done by the implant manufacturer McGhan, after three years, 39 percent of reconstruction patients needed additional surgical treatment and 23 percent had implants removed. This company's studies also show that after three years, 21 percent of augmentation patients had additional surgical treatment and 8 percent had them removed. Even though women with augmentation with saline implants have fewer complications and the newer saline implants are stronger, the IOM report concluded that 18 percent of women with modern saline implants for augmentation suffered a local complication within one year, and 36 percent of those who had reconstruction suffered complications within one year.

In an interview with *Glamour* magazine in November 2000, Norman Anderson, M.D., former chair of the FDA's medical-devices committee and currently associate professor of medicine at Johns Hopkins School of Medicine, said, "These are shocking data." He tried to stop the FDA from approving saline implants and testified that saline implants "have the potential to have the highest failure rate of any device ever approved by the FDA." He said some of his patients have had as many as fourteen operations to replace failed saline implants. (The FDA has published photos of complications of breast implants on the web at: http://www.fda. gov/cdrh/breastimplants/breast_implants_photos.html)

Implant surgery carries with it the usual known risks and complications of any major surgery—bleeding, infection, delayed wound healing, pain, and reactions to anesthesia, to name the primary ones. Local complications are often serious enough so that many women need to have additional medical attention, and this often means additional surgeries to remove or replace the implants. This puts them at further risk for general surgical complications, and ironically it may also lead to more local complications. According to Diana Zuckerman, Ph.D., "There's a growing body of research that shows that women who have had implants a second or third or more times tend to have more complications than women who have had them once."

Three things are certain:

◆ It is highly likely that anyone with implants will have at least one local complication.

- The risk of having a local complication increases the older your implant gets.

- Implants do not last forever, and women with implants will almost certainly require at least one replacement surgery during their lifetime, and sometimes several—perhaps every eight to ten years.

## Capsular Contracture

As a natural reaction to something foreign, such as an implant, being inserted into it, the body forms a protective membrane of scar tissue around the object. This layer of tissue normally shrinks to some degree against the implant. However, in a number of women with breast implants, the protective mechanism is overenthusiastic. The scar tissue builds up, and the capsule of scar tissue may tighten too much (contract). This contracture squeezes the implant, and, as a result, the breast feels firmer and may be uncomfortable. In severe cases the contracture is quite painful and causes a misshapen appearance. Some women are unable to sleep on their abdomens because of their rock-hard breasts. Others are self-conscious during close physical contact, even friendly hugging. The "tennis ball effect" can also cause the implant to move upward, making it quite obvious that the woman's breasts are not hers—they are implants—when the woman is nude or wearing certain types of revealing clothing.

In 1992 the FDA advisory panel found that the percentage of women who experienced contracture was not known, but estimates range from 10 percent to as high as 70 percent. Since then, we have learned a bit more, although we still have a lot more to learn. Studies of saline implants by the implant manufacturers show that after one year, 5–7 percent of augmentation patients and 13–29 percent of reconstruction patients had capsular contracture. At three years, the figures were 9 percent and 25–30 percent respectively. When silicone and saline implants were compared in women who had undergone reconstruction, one study showed that 54 percent of the women receiving silicone-gel implants had contractures of classes III and IV after only six months (see sidebar for a description of classes).

It seems that contracture progresses and worsens over time, and that each time it is treated, the treatment is less successful. Of those who had their implants removed and replaced, after two years 7 percent of augmentation patients had class III or IV contracture again, and 48 percent of reconstruction patients had contracture again. According to a 1999 report, class III and IV contractures reach 100 percent around silicone-gel-filled implants at twenty-five years. Other studies show that, overall, 73 percent of the implants removed were due to contracture. In women with augmented breasts, 28 percent of the additional procedures were due to this complication; in women with reconstructed breasts, the proportion was 14 percent.

We don't know why some women suffer severe contractures and others don't, but plastic surgeons have many theories and keep fine-tuning their surgical and postsurgical techniques in an effort to prevent it. There is some evidence that saline implants cause less contracture than silicone gel, and that in some women textured implants cause less contracture than smooth ones. Also, positioning the implant behind the chest muscle rather than above it may lessen the degree and incidence of contracture. Some researchers, including Canadian Pierre Blais, think that contracture is caused by body fluids entering the implant—possibly through

> **CLASSES OF CONTRACTURE**
>
> The degree of capsular contracture is measured on a scale called the Baker Classification:
>
> **Class I** The implanted breast is still as soft as a nonimplanted breast
>
> **Class II** The implanted breast is less soft, and the implant can be felt, but is not visible
>
> **Class III** The implanted breast is firmer and the implant can be felt easily as well as seen, or the breast looks distorted
>
> **Class IV** The breast is firm, hard, tender, and painful, and it is markedly distorted

the valves or through the envelope—causing the implant to expand and the scar capsule to become tighter and harder. (This phenomenon may also explain why implants often contain blood and other body fluids, as well as why bacteria and fungi can grow inside a "sterile" saline solution.) Dr. Susan Kolb, a plastic surgeon, believes contractures may be the result of a low-grade infection around the implant, possibly due to the presence of bacteria in the breast ducts, to which the implants are exposed when they are placed above the muscle. The IOM report concludes that contracture may be more common if a hematoma (collection of blood) or seroma (collection of the watery portion of the blood) is present in the breast.

Although contracture is not a health hazard in and of itself, it can cause debilitating pain and lead to serious additional complications, including repeated operations in an attempt to correct the condition. A patient may undergo surgery to break up the fibrous tissue or to remove it, and sometimes it is necessary to remove and replace the implant. Of course, the additional surgery carries additional risks, such as infection, reaction to the anesthesia, and scarring. The surgery may also involve removing some breast tissue along with the entire hardened scar capsule.

Melvin Spira, professor of surgery in the Division of Plastic Surgery at the Baylor College of Medicine, says:

> We now know a number of things about the implants that we perhaps didn't know twenty years ago. For example, some women do form a very firm capsule, and some of them do have pain. We used to feel if there was a problem it was due to surgeon error or patient noncompliance. We now feel—at least I do very strongly—that there are a very small number of women who are adversely affected by their implants—either silicone-gel or saline—and we should not keep repeating the same operation over and over again, taking the implant and the capsule out, putting another implant back in again. I would say the implant should be left out permanently.

Some experts theorize that contracture may pose another health hazard: It may squeeze the implant so tightly that the implant ruptures or extrudes through the skin. (The potential harm

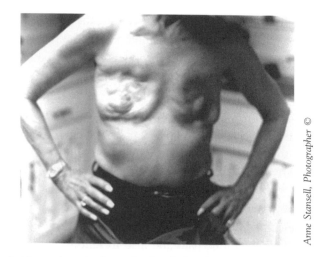

*Anne Stansell, Photographer ©*

*When deciding to have implants, decide whether the possible benefits are worth the possible consequences. Surgeons show photos of their best results (and sometimes the beautiful results of other surgeons). It is not likely that they will show you photos like this one. This woman's husband convinced her to have breast implants. Five years later, she says, the surgeons removed what was left of her ruptured implants, which required removing damaged breast tissue as well as removing silicone from her ribs, back, and collarbone area. In addition to these local complications, she also became sick with heart problems, mental confusion, and neurological damage. She says, "my husband could not deal with my constant illness and he left me."*

from rupture is discussed later in this chapter.) This is the reason that a "closed capsulotomy"—wherein the surgeon exerts strong pressure on the breast to force the scar tissue to soften—is no longer recommended as treatment. Such a procedure can be very painful, and it can rupture the implant while giving only temporary relief from the complication, if any.

Contracture also affects the ability to detect breast cancer, either by physical exam or by mammography. See page 82 for a full discussion of implants and cancer detection. Dr. Neal Handel believes that insurance companies should consider surgical correction of contracture "medically necessary" because of the pain, deformity, and detrimental effect it has on cancer detection.

Here is what it was like for one woman who experienced contracture after reconstruction:

> I've had problems with silicone implants for years. I have
> small breasts and the first implant was too big; I had it
> replaced with another, but it was too big, too. I then had a
> third one custom-made, and I had a good result for a while,
> but after a couple of years it was so contracted. It had moved
> upward on my chest so that you could tell when I wore thin
> clothing such as a silk blouse. Also, the bottom part of my
> breast had dimpled in. I was so embarrassed that I'd sit in
> the hot tub with my husband, but not my friends. I was dis-
> satisfied, but I didn't know anyone else with implants, and I
> thought, "Well, you've had cancer—you shouldn't expect to
> look perfect."

## Rupture and Deflation

Another extremely common complication occurs when the envelope breaks or sustains a hole or tear, allowing the contents to spill
outside the envelope. The implant's outer envelope may break due
to trauma or injury (such as in a car accident) or normal wear and
aging. In the past, such trauma was often caused by a nonsurgical
procedure called *closed capsulotomy*, formerly (but no longer) used
to break up hard scar tissue around the implant. Rupture may also
be caused by small imperfections in the envelope, or may occur
during the initial implant surgery when the surgeon stitches the
incision closed. An implant may also be punctured during a needle biopsy. Saline implants may leak because of defective or
unsealed valves.

Dr. Susan Kolb points to evidence that the body itself may
weaken the silicone shell, by "punching holes in the silicone" and
allowing the contents eventually to spill out. During this process,
called *lipolysis*, the body's enzymes break down the silicone, and
immune cells called *macrophages* engulf or "eat" the silicone. "The
same implant put on a shelf will not disintegrate," she says. The

macrophages then travel to other parts of the body with their toxic payload, but that is a story to explore in the next chapter.

When a saline implant ruptures, the implant generally deflates within a couple of days. The implant shell simply collapses, like a water balloon, and the contents are easily absorbed by the body. Rarely, a saline implant may develop a small, slow leak that takes one or two years to notice. Saline-implant ruptures are therefore usually quite obvious and require immediate removal and replacement to maintain the augmented or reconstructed appearance.

This is not the case with silicone-gel implants; ruptures or leaks in silicone-gel-filled implants usually are detected only quite a bit later, and, often, not until the implant has been surgically removed. Most of the major health concerns about implants relate to ruptured silicone-gel implants. Rupture of a silicone-gel-filled implant would allow the gel to escape and possibly seep into the surrounding tissue or migrate to other parts of the body.

A rupture in a silicone-gel implant can be *intracapsular* (when the scar capsule surrounding the implant stays intact, containing

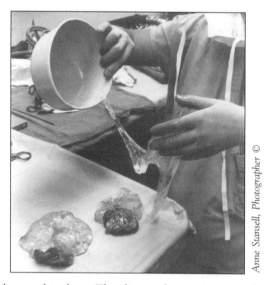

Anne Stansell, Photographer ©

*Ruptured silicone-gel implants. The silicone gel may migrate to other parts of the body, such as the arms, groin, nerves, lung, and internal organs.*

the gel—at least for the time being) or *extracapsular* (when the scar capsule breaks and the gel escapes into nearby tissue and perhaps migrates to distant tissue). Gel from broken implants may migrate outside the capsule and create lumps called *granulomas* in the nearby chest tissue. Silicone lumps may also occur in the arm, the armpit, and even farther afield. In some women, free silicone causes lymph nodes in the armpits to enlarge, a condition called *lymphadenopathy*.

Some surgeons, such as Loren Eskenazi, feel that "unless you have symptoms, you don't need to worry if the shell dissolves or ruptures, because everyone has a small amount of gel bleed in the implant capsule anyway" (bleed is described later in this chapter). However, she states, "Extracapsular rupture is another story; this is the equivalent of having silicone injected directly into your breasts." Others believe that any ruptured gel implant needs to come out. Paul Striker, also a plastic surgeon, says:

> Once the implant has lost its integrity, the silicone is going to get out. If there's nothing to hold the silicone, then your body is going to wall it off again, inside the capsule; smaller subcapsules will form, and you'll get lumps and more spherical capsular contraction. The scar tissue may be soft or thin; it might be too flimsy to hold free silicone. With pressure, silicone could extrude through the scar, or if there's a rent in the capsule, nodules of silicone can go through tissue planes to distant areas…into the axilla [armpits], down into the groin, the legs, rib cage, the nerves of the arm—those are the real complications of ruptured implants.

Striker gives the example of a woman who has pain in her fingers: "We might find a lump in the armpit; when we take it out, we find it's a silicone granule." Another patient fell while she was ice skating. She noticed a lump in her groin a few months later and thought she had cancer, but it turned out to be a silicone granule. Striker explains that because these granules are relatively large amounts of silicone as far as the body is concerned, "they don't get metabolized; the body has to wall them off."

In 1992, the FDA found that the percentage of implants that rupture is "uncertain," but that the rupture rate may be higher than previously thought. How right they were. Finding straight answers about the frequency of ruptures still isn't easy, especially with gel implants, because they do not so obviously deflate. In reviewing the studies available up to 1999, the IOM concluded that "risks accumulate over the lifetime of the implant, but quantitative data on this point are lacking for modern implants and are deficient historically." The University of Florida also did its own analysis of thirty-five implant studies, which was published in 1999. These researchers concluded that silicone-breast-implant rupture rates were approximately 30 percent after five years, 50 percent after ten years, and 70 percent at seventeen years. According to some reports, saline-filled implants have a higher incidence of failure than gel-filled types. But Dr. Striker believes saline implants have gotten a bad rap. "I've had very few leakages over the years," he says. "The rate of leakage depends a lot on the model. Some early models had valves that were defective, but medical advances have been made, and now the track record is much better."

We still don't know if Striker is right. Although saline implants have improved, and those being used today appear to have a deflation rate of up to 3 percent after the first year and 5 to 10 percent after ten years, we have no data beyond the ten-year point. In one study, in which women were followed for an average of six years, 10 percent had at least one deflated implant. Mentor's three-year study shows a deflation rate of 3 percent for augmented patients and 9 percent for reconstruction patients; McGhan's three-year studies found a 5 percent and 6 percent deflation rate, respectively.

A patient who has a ruptured silicone implant may notice decreased breast size, hard lumps, changes in the appearance of the breast, pain or tenderness, tingling, swelling, numbness, burning, or changes in sensation. But she may also experience a "silent rupture," one with no symptoms. Ruptures—particularly intracapsular ones—can be difficult to detect, even with mammography;

in fact, some experts feel mammography is another possible source of trauma to the implant. Ultrasound or magnetic resonance imaging (MRI) may be used to detect or confirm broken implants in some cases.

Michael Middleton, a radiologist at the University of California, San Diego, perfected the MRI scan to show silicone in the body. He recently participated in an FDA study published in 2000. The study included 344 women who'd gotten their first implants before 1988. Between them, they had a total of 687 silicone-gel implants. They were given MRIs, and Middleton and his coauthors concluded that 55 percent of the implants had ruptured—this translates into 69 percent of the women (some women had more than one implant). Another 7 percent had implants that were "suspicious." This means that the majority of the women in the study—76 percent—had at least one breast implant that was rated by these experts as ruptured or probably ruptured. Of the 344 women, 21 percent had extracapsular silicone gel in one or both breasts. They estimated that the median age of the implant when it ruptured was 10.8 years. They concluded that "The prevalence of silent or occult silicone gel implant rupture is higher than previously suspected." This study also found that rupture is linked with a higher incidence of fibromyalgia; the finding that rupture is both silent and is more likely the longer a woman has an implant may be why other studies don't show an increase in systemic disease.

Another study of three hundred women who had silicone-gel implants for one to twenty-five years and then had them removed found similar results. The researchers saw visible signs of shell rupture in 51 percent of the women; severe silicone leakage (with no visible tears or holes in the shells) was found in an additional 20 percent. Other studies show extracapsular rupture in 11 to 23 percent of women.

As is the case with saline implants, the age of the implant and the year it was made are factors. Silicone-gel implants made between 1975 and 1986 have a higher rate of leaking and rupture because the envelopes were made with thinner walls and contained

a thinner, more fluid silicone gel. The FDA says these earlier models "may have excessively leaked silicone gel and may not have
been tested adequately."

Middleton's data on the relative risk of rupture in specific types
of implants, which he compiled with coauthor M. K. Dobke, were
first published in 1994. He says that "roughly, the implants are
running neck and neck. The exception is the polyurethane-coated
implant—the risk is much worse." In his experience, the rupture
or leak rate of a ten- to twelve-year-old non-polyurethane-coated
implant is 10 to 15 percent. The rupture or leak rate of a
polyurethane-coated implant of the same age is 100 percent. At
ten years, the rate is 8 percent for uncoated implants, and 80 percent for coated implants. However, this is inconsistent with the
FDA study that found very high rupture rates even though it did
not include polyurethane-coated implants. Middleton feels strongly
that a number of implants suffer from microruptures—tiny leaks
in a degraded shell—that allow gel to get out in addition to oil
(silicone liquid mixed with silicone gel, which acts as a lubricant).
He feels that most physicians "have no appreciation that this problem exists, or that it may affect the patient, which it probably does."

Melvin Spira acknowledges, "We used to think they were
almost fail-safe, but they're not. Breast implants are devices and
all have the potential for failure." There are always exceptions.
Spira says he was in the operating room when the first silicone-gel
implant was placed, in 1962. "This woman is still doing well." Of
course, she had an early implant, with a thicker, stronger envelope
and gel. However, in general, for both types of implants, time is a
factor: Several studies suggest that the longer a woman has an
implant, the greater the chance of leaks and ruptures. Many surgeons believe that any implant over ten years old is likely to be
leaking or ruptured.

The two women's stories that follow illustrate the differences
between a ruptured silicone implant and a ruptured saline implant:

> ◆    I got my silicone implants in 1978 and they hardened
> almost immediately. That never bothered me, really. What
> bothered me was the increasing controversy over their safety.

I went to see a plastic surgeon about doing a totally unrelated cosmetic procedure and we happened to talk about my
implants. He said, "You've got a pair of dinosaurs in there"—
that's how old they were. He then put a saline implant and a
gel implant on a piece of paper. When he picked them up, I
saw how stained the paper was from the silicone bleeding
through the shell. That's when I started giving serious
thought to having my implants removed.

Next I had a sonogram, but it didn't detect anything
wrong. My mammogram had shown nothing, too. But all my
doctors were advising me to remove them, even so. I finally
scheduled the surgery, but then agonized for the next six
weeks: "Why am I putting myself through this? There's a
tremendous risk in removing them—and then I'll have to
recover from surgery on top of it all!"

Fortunately, I went through with it. The three-hour surgery took over five hours. My implants had ruptured, and my
surgeon told me his fingers were black and blue from all the
work it took to clean the gel out. We still don't know why
nothing showed on the sonogram, but I am one lucky woman.

◆   Before my surgery, my surgeon told me about a patient of
his whose implants had deflated from the force on her chest
during a car accident. Since she had saline implants, there
were no problems with the gel afterward. Still, I never
thought it would happen to me. But it did. One night, about
three years after my implants were put in, I was doing the
squeezing exercises my surgeon showed me to keep the
implants soft. I noticed my left breast was different. I thought,
"Uh-oh, something is wrong here." And I freaked out! I was
frightened, shocked. So many things were running through
my head. Fortunately, I reached my doctor right away and he
calmed me down. He said this is why he used saline—just in
case something like this happened. The deflation wasn't physically uncomfortable at all, but I was self-conscious about the
way it looked. Not that it looked horrible—but the skin had
stretched to accommodate the implant, it was a little smaller,
and it drooped. It wasn't deformed or anything. I just wore
loose clothing for the next two weeks until my surgery to
replace it.

## Gel Bleed and Shedding

Even if an implant does not actually rupture or have an obvious leak, we now know that most silicone-gel implants allow small amounts of silicone to seep out through the covering. This is called *gel bleed*. At one point plastic surgeons pressured implant manufacturers to make thinner envelopes in order to keep the breast softer. However, this not only increased the risk of implant rupture; it also allowed for more gel bleed. Manufacturers have since changed their design, and implants made after the mid-'80s have envelopes designed to reduce gel bleed.

The authors of *Women's Health Alert* equate gel bleed with "repeated small injections of silicone." An FDA memo asserts that even these small, gradual leaks pose a serious risk and may result in deposition and migration of silicone in the body, leading to capsular contracture, granuloma, and enlarged lymph nodes. It also appears that the implant shell can shed silicone particles. Implant ruptures, leaks, bleed, and shedding are all suspect in causing the serious systemic problems described in Chapter 5.

## Unsatisfactory Appearance

After implant surgery, some women may dislike the way they look. Implants can wrinkle, be placed incorrectly (too high, too low, off to one side), or have a sloshing sound and feel. Implant recipients may sustain wide, raised, or otherwise noticeable scarring. They may not like the size or shape of their new breast. They may be able to feel or see the valve in a saline implant. Additional surgery can correct some of these undesirable outcomes, but additional surgery may also create more. In the three-year McGhan studies, 6 to 11 percent of the augmentation patients experienced problems with appearance due to wrinkling, asymmetry, ability to feel or see the implants, implants in the wrong position, and scarring. Reconstruction patients fared worse: 33 percent experienced moderate, severe, or very severe asymmetry; 23 percent experienced wrinkling, or the ability to see or feel the implant; 12 percent experienced improper positioning of the implant; and 6 percent had bad scarring.

## Infection

Patients may develop an infection in the surgical area. This requires additional medical treatment, such as antibiotics, or perhaps surgery to remove or replace the implant. Women who have had reconstruction appear to be most at risk for local infections, especially after immediate reconstruction. Some studies suggest that some women sustain "subclinical" infections around the implants, which are unable to be detected or reached by antibiotics. The implants, which are the source of the infection, must be removed before these women can be treated successfully. Pain is often a sign of infection, and in these cases, antibiotic therapy and replacement with sterile implants usually relieves the pain. Bacterial infections are thought to be a possible contributor to capsular contraction. Local infections can spread throughout the body, and some experts believe this may be one factor in the systemic disease from which women with implants suffer. According to Dr. Susan Kolb, "We see infection more in textured implants than in smooth ones. And silicone-gel implants have about 50 percent positive cultures, and the textured saline have about 95 percent positive cultures. So it's serious."

Many researchers have been looking at implant-related infection. Dr. Pierre Blais, Ph.D., a former scientific advisor for Health Canada's Health Protection Branch, has analyzed over seven thousand implants and has found various types of fungus, algae, and antibiotic-resistant bacteria. Dr. V. Leroy Young, professor of plastic surgery at Washington University in St. Louis, has demonstrated that E. coli, staph, and aspergillus fungus can grow in saline implants. Dr. Marek Dobke, M.D., head of the division of plastic surgery at the University of California, San Diego, School of Medicine, examined implants removed from three hundred women who had complained of the systemic symptoms discussed in the next chapter. He found bacteria or fungi in about 70 percent of these women, which was three times the incidence of infection in women without symptoms; he also confirmed the association between contamination and capsular contracture and pain.

Obviously, immediately post-op is a high-risk time for local infection around an implant. But, says Dr. Neal Handel, "Some women can do well for years, and then suddenly have acute swelling and fluid in the breast. When we culture it, we don't find anything, but most people think it's either due to a viral infection or an organism that doesn't grow in the culture." How does the organism get there, years after someone has been all sewn up and healed? "Through the circulatory system," says Handel. "Bacteria could get into your system from an infection in another part of your body, such as a urinary tract infection, and colonize the surface of the implant. The area of the implant has less resistance to infection—white blood cells and antibodies and other infection-fighting components of the immune system can't get to the implant and that's why they are always at some risk of getting infected."

## Pain and Other Changes in Breast Sensation

Few studies about implants have looked at pain, yet it is one of the more frequent reasons why women have their implants replaced or removed. Pain related to implants can be severe and can occur after surgery and persist for many days or weeks, particularly after reconstruction. Pain may be the result of nerve compression, nerve damage, capsular contracture, interference with muscle motion, or improper surgical technique. Pain may also indicate a bacterial infection or silicone-gel-implant rupture.

In addition, implant surgery may increase or decrease the sensitivity of the breast or nipple. This change may be temporary or permanent. Such changes may occur because nerves are cut, especially if the surgeon makes the incision through the nipple. Or they may be due to stretching of the nerves caused by the presence of the implant, particularly if the breasts were very small and a relatively large implant was inserted.

These changes in sensation can interfere with sexual enjoyment, sexual response, and one's ability to nurse a baby.

Studies show that up to half of women endure substantial pain after reconstruction, and up to 38 percent have pain after augmentation. The pain may begin immediately after surgery; it may subside, or it may linger. Many women (about 20 to 29 percent) with pain require pain medication.

The McGhan three-year study of saline implants found that 16 percent of women with augmentation experienced breast pain, 9 percent had intense nipple sensation, 8 percent had loss of nipple sensation, and 7 percent had intense skin sensations. In reconstruction patients, the percentages were similar, except 15 percent experienced breast pain and 12 percent lost nipple sensation at three years. In the McGhan three-year studies, 10 percent of augmentation patients experienced loss of nipple sensation, 5 percent experienced intense nipple sensation, and 5 percent experienced breast pain; in these studies, 35 percent of reconstruction patients lost nipple sensation and 17 percent experienced breast pain. Dr. Diana Zuckerman believes that loss of nipple sensation is probably underreported. As an example, she sites the McGhan study, in which 35 percent of the reconstructed women reported that they lost nipple sensation; however, she points out that it is unlikely that these women have nipples or much breast sensation at all, so the percentage is likely closer to 100 percent. She feels this effect may similarly be underreported in augmentation patients as well.

## Calcium Deposits

In some women, calcium forms in the tissue surrounding the silicone-gel or saline-filled implant. Like capsular contracture, this may cause hardening and pain. Since microcalcification is a possible indicator of early breast cancer, calcium deposits caused by implants may raise unnecessary alarm, and implant removal and/or unnecessary biopsies may be performed to determine whether the deposits are cancer related. The cause of calcification is unknown, but it appears to be part of the process of scar formation, and the risk varies according to an individual's biochemistry. Loren Eskenazi observes that calcification is more common in women with older implants.

## Interference with Mammography and Cancer Detection

There is concern that both silicone-gel and saline-filled implants can decrease the chance of early detection of breast cancer and thus lessen the chance for a cure. Now that so many women with implants are reaching their forties and fifties—the age at which the risk of breast cancer begins to rise—it is critical that we understand the impact breast implants could have on the ability to detect breast cancer early. This issue is currently being studied and hotly debated. The IOM report concluded that no studies of women with breast implants have shown increases in deaths from breast cancer because the diagnosis was delayed. However, it also concluded that this issue needs to be studied further.

Currently, two main methods exist for detecting breast cancer: physically examining the breasts for palpable lumps and mammography. Physical exams usually detect cancers that are two centimeters or larger (about four-fifths of an inch). Such cancers are usually about five to seven years old and are not "early cancers" because they have had a long time in which to spread. Consequently, by the time they are found, about half of these cancers have already spread to the lymph nodes in the armpit; only about 60 to 80 percent of women at this stage live another five years.

Mammography lets us detect cancers earlier, long before lumps are detectable by feel. Just 5 percent of the smallest cancers detected by mammogram have spread to the lymph nodes, and the five-year survival rate ranges from 90 to 95 percent. Although a five-year survival should by no means be considered a "cure," the higher percentage gives mammograms the edge. While mammography is controversial and certainly not fail-proof nor a guarantee, it presents the possibility of detecting breast cancer at a more curable stage and is the best tool we have at this time.

Neal Handel, a plastic surgeon formerly with the Van Nuys Breast Center, and his colleagues, surgeon Melvin Silverstein and radiologist Parvis Gamagami, have conducted several studies on the effect of breast implants on mammography and breast cancer detection. They and other researchers—such as V. Leroy Young and his colleagues at the Washington University School of Medicine in St. Louis—have found that implants can affect mammography by implant "shadow," tissue compression, and in several other ways.

## Implant "Shadow"

All implants are radiopaque: They block the mammography X-ray beam as it passes through the breast, obscuring the tissue in front of and behind the prosthesis (and creating a "shadow" of the implant on the film). As a result, small tumors remain hidden and undiagnosed. The silicone shell itself interferes slightly—more so if it is folded or twisted, which occurs most often after a saline or double-lumen implant deflates or a gel implant ruptures. But the implant filler is the main culprit. Studies using animals, "mammographic phantoms," cadavers, and women volunteers have shown that silicone gel obscures almost everything in front of and behind it; saline obscures less, and peanut oil least of all. (An implant made of soybean oil was developed and tested, but was withdrawn because of massive problems with implant failure. See Chapter 3.)

The Van Nuys group found that the degree of capsular contracture was the primary factor determining how much breast tissue could be seen in a mammogram conducted on a woman with implants. In women with mild contracture, they could see about 70 percent of the breast, but with moderate or severe contraction, only 50 percent of the breast showed. Young cites studies that have shown that silicone and saline implants obscured 22 percent to 83 percent of the breast tissue during a mammogram.

## Tissue Compression

Breast implants mechanically squeeze the surrounding breast tissue. This increases tissue density and makes it difficult to detect

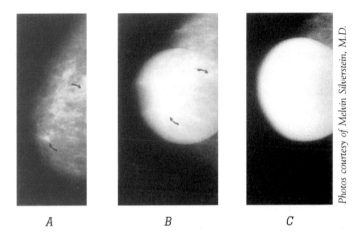

*Photos courtesy of Melvin Silverstein, M.D.*

|  A  |  B  |  C  |

*The effect of different materials on the ability of a mammogram to visualize the presence of known abnormalities: (A) Baseline mammogram. The upper arrow points to microcalcifications; the lower arrow points to a soft-tissue mass. Both lesions (abnormalities) are clearly seen. (B) Mammogram of a saline-filled implant. The image is less clear than the baseline mammogram. (C) Mammogram of a silicone-gel-filled implant. The lesions cannot be seen at all.*

small abnormalities and subtle distortions in a mammogram, which are often the first clues to breast cancer.

In addition, the very presence of the implant makes it difficult to compress tissue adequately during mammography. Flattening of the breast tissue creates a thinner, wider layer for the X rays to penetrate, making it much easier to see tiny lumps or suspicious abnormalities. Dr. Handel explains that "whereas the average nonaugmented breast can be compressed to a thickness of 4.5 centimeters during mammography, the augmented breast can typically be compressed to a thickness of only 7 centimeters," resulting in a less readable mammogram. And contracture worsens the picture. The greater the capsular contracture, the denser the surrounding tissue, resulting in a less clear mammographic image that is harder to interpret.

## Other Effects of Implants on Mammograms

The surgery to insert and remove implants causes scarring. This in turn may lead to distortions, densities, and calcifications visible on the mammogram or felt during a physical exam. Benign abnormalities may be confused with cancer; cancerous abnormalities may be assumed to be benign. Textured implants pose another problem, since the surface may fill with tissue and mimic a rupture or other abnormality on the X-ray film.

Some women who have implants for reconstruction have surgery performed on the healthy breast (see pages 53 and 61) so that it better matches the reconstructed breast. This scarring can also confuse the mammogram, causing a great deal of uncertainty in women who are already at higher than usual risk for breast cancer.

The first time my radiologist told me about the microcalcifications in my healthy breast I was blasé—confident that it was just the scarring from the uplift. But he insisted on doing extra mammograms to magnify the suspicious area. Back I went, my heart in my throat until I got the "all clear." Now I routinely get the magnifications—along with an extra dose of radiation, which doesn't thrill me. What if all that extra radiation eventually causes another breast cancer? This is a possibility, although my doctors agree the danger is slight compared with the danger of missing an early cancer. Small comfort that the mammogram would detect a cancer that it may itself have created.

Neal Handel and his colleagues believe that the above factors explain why, in the patients they studied, women who have breast cancer after augmentation are diagnosed at a later stage than women without implants: Their diagnosis is delayed due to their implants. Between 1981 and 1992, the Breast Center treated fifty-two women with augmented breasts who had developed breast cancer, and 1,550 breast cancer patients without implants. The center found significant differences between the two groups regarding tumor size, spread to lymph nodes, and length of survival. For example, mammography missed tumors in 42 percent of the augmented women with palpable lumps. In contrast, mammography missed tumors in only 8 percent of the nonaugmented women with palpable lumps. In another study, published in 1993, Douglas Reintgen, of the University of South Florida in Tampa, reported that five out of eight palpable breast cancers went undetected by mammography in women with augmented breasts. Dr. Handel has seen women with palpable breast cancer that was invisible on a mammogram, but this occurs even without implants.

Not everyone agrees with the findings of the Van Nuys or Tampa groups. A Canadian study by Dale Birdsell, for instance, does not support their findings. Birdsell and his colleagues compared 41 women who developed breast cancer after augmentation with 13,246 women who had breast cancer but not implants. They found that the tumors in women with implants were smaller than those in other women, although the incidence of spreading to the lymph nodes and other sites was equal. The five- and ten-year survival rates were also comparable, even though the women with implants were diagnosed at a younger age. (Other studies show that younger women—under forty—tend to die sooner after diagnosis than women diagnosed at age forty and over.) The researchers concluded that breast augmentation is not a cause for concern in diagnosing breast cancer.

Handel admits that these conflicting results are "a bone of contention between us and other researchers." He refers to other data published by Dennis Deapan and Garry Brody, of the University of Southern California (see "Cancer" in Chapter 5), suggesting that the incidence of cancer is not any higher—in fact it is lower—in women with implants, and that the stage of disease is the same in augmented as in nonaugmented patients. These two researchers are also conducting an ongoing epidemiological survey of all women in Los Angeles County. They are looking at all stages of breast cancer—from very early in situ precancer to advanced cancer—and have found that the percentages are basically the same whether the women have implants or not. Thus, this is a piece of evidence that suggests that implants do not interfere with the diagnosis of breast cancer at any stage.

"Our answer to that," Handel says, "is that most of the patients are being diagnosed with palpable breast cancer—in other words, it's relatively advanced compared to what mammography is capable of diagnosing. We don't feel implants will interfere significantly with the diagnosis of palpable breast cancer, but we do feel that they will interfere with occult [hidden] breast cancer"—and the purpose of mammography is to find occult cancers. "You need to find tumors long before they can be felt—five, seven, eight years before," Handel continues. He believes that although the USC studies show no detrimental effect of implants on cancer detection, "to us that just means women are not having good-quality mammography frequently enough. The important point to make is that breast implants are going to interfere with the early detection of cancer, not the late detection." He points to another ongoing study at UCLA that is showing similar findings to his own study—"that it was harder to find cancer in augmented women and it is being found at a later stage." And another cause for concern is a 2002 NIH-based study by lead investigator Louise Brinton; it found that cancers were diagnosed at a more advanced stage in augmented women.

As you will see in Chapter 6, special mammography techniques were developed in 1988 that allow specially trained technicians to do mammograms with less compression of the implant, and that show more tissue than regular mammography does. However, these techniques require more views to be taken, and this increases a woman's exposure to radiation, which is a known cause of cancer.

## Other Local Complications

Women with implants should be aware of several other possible local complications.

### Hematoma/Seroma

Sometimes blood or serum (the watery portion of the blood) collects at the surgery site; these complications are called *hematoma* and *seroma*, respectively. They may contribute to infection, capsular contraction, or both. The patient may experience swelling, bruising, and pain. The body may be able to absorb the accumulated fluid, but some patients must be drained to heal properly.

## Necrosis

Necrosis is the death of the tissue around the implant. It may prevent proper wound healing and require additional surgery or removal of the implant. A sufferer of necrosis may be permanently scarred or may lose tissue, leaving her breast deformed. Infection, smoking, and insertion of steroids in the implant pocket are associated with increased risk of necrosis.

## Breast-Tissue Atrophy or Chest-Wall Deformity

Breast implants exert pressure on nearby tissues; this can cause the tissue to atrophy—that is, to get thinner or to waste away—resulting in a deformity of the chest wall. It may occur while a woman still has implants, or it may be noticeable only after they are removed.

## Galactorrhea

Breast-implant surgery can cause a woman to begin spontaneously producing breast milk, an occurrence known as *galactorrhea*. The condition might stop by itself, or the patient may need to take medication that suppresses milk production. Some women must have their breast implants removed because they continue to produce milk.

# 5

# Effects of Implants on the Whole Body (Systemic Disease)

In addition to the relatively well recognized (if still incompletely understood) local effects discussed in Chapter 4, questions have been raised about whether breast implants can cause serious systemic disease. This is the most hotly debated area of the silicone-implant controversy. The questions mostly surround the gel filler, but since the envelope itself is also made of silicone, questions exist about saline implants as well. Since the FDA ruling in 1992, a dedicated and growing number of researchers and clinicians have been developing and refining theories as to why and how silicone could provoke a body-wide response, and through diligent experimentation they are slowly unraveling silicone's secrets. However, it is still far from clear what the silicone-related disease is, how common it is, who is at higher risk, why it occurs, how to diagnose it, and how to treat it. We don't even have an accepted name for "it" or know whether more than one type of disease exists. In addition, there may be separate issues that have to do with chemical contaminants and with saline implants regarding local and system-wide bacterial and fungal infections and their effects on the entire body. So, perhaps the best name at this time is "breast-implant disease."

Although some women's symptoms resemble classic and painful connective-tissue and autoimmune disorders such as fibromyalgia (muscle weakness and pain), rheumatoid arthritis (crippling, painful, swollen joints), and scleroderma (painful hardening of the skin and organs), some researchers believe that women are experiencing an entirely new and unique syndrome related specifically to silicone. Like AIDS, chronic fatigue syndrome, and environmental illness/multiple chemical sensitivities, silicone-related disease may belong to an emerging group of puzzling diseases we have never seen before.

Dr. Susan Kolb, an Atlanta plastic surgeon who is also board certified in holistic medicine, is one of many female plastic surgeons who have had silicone breast implants. However, she is, to her knowledge and to mine, the only one who has gotten sick with silicone disease and has admitted it. Because of her holistic training, and because she has treated over a thousand sick women who have implants, she thinks "outside the box." She says, "We are nowhere near to understanding this disease. It is a giant experiment. It is a newly emerging disease."

In addition to immune disorders and chemical poisoning, there is concern that silicone implants could cause or influence the progression of cancer, or cause birth defects and other adverse effects in children of women with implants.

## Interactions Between Silicone and the Immune System

The immune system is part of a larger defense system designed to protect us from disease and foreign invaders. Many substances in our environment—such as metals, pesticides, and air pollution—interfere with our immune system's activity. Such substances may suppress or put our immune system into overdrive, conditions that each have their own symptoms and make us more susceptible to disease. Exposure to certain substances may lead to autoimmune disease, wherein our immune system mistakenly attacks our own cells, destroying healthy tissue. It is believed that in rheumatic dis-eases the immune system attacks muscles, joints, nerves, connec-tive tissue, and bones.

It was once thought that silicone was biologically inert—that it had no effect on the cells of the body. In retrospect, one has to wonder: How could we think we could put silicone in the body for ten, twenty, thirty years, and the body wasn't going to react?

"That's absolutely right," agrees Harry Spiera, a rheumatolo-gist at the Mount Sinai School of Medicine and one of the first to report possible autoimmune effects from implants. "Over the course of two million years nature evolved an immune system to get rid of infection and foreign material, and I think it's hubris to put this stuff in and think it's not going to do anything. We know that sil-icone wrist implants break down and dissolve the surrounding bone. The lesson is: there's a difference between being chemically inert and biologically inert."

Some people may react to silicone more strongly than others, or sooner, or to smaller amounts. We've already seen in Chapter 4 that the body reacts to an implant as a foreign body, encasing it in scar tissue (encapsulization). This scar tissue was once thought to completely protect the body from further exposure to silicone. Though we have long known that silicone implants bleed, it was thought that even if silicone particles entered the capsule wall, they remained trapped. It is now apparent that silicone particles escape through the capsule and travel to other parts of the body, including lymph nodes in the armpits and neck; the liver; and the lungs. As Saul Puzskin, professor of pathology at the Mount Sinai School of Medicine, describes it, "The scar is made of fibrous tis-sue—it's not solid really. It's like layer after layer of fishing net that acts like a filter. The silicone moves slowly like a current through it."

Thus the likelihood of silicone migration exists not only (as was previously thought) when there is a rupture and large amounts are forced out of the breast capsule and into nearby tissue, or after silicone has been directly injected into the breasts. The slow, steady bleed of even an intact silicone-gel implant exposes the immune system to silicone. There is evidence that the silicone shell also sheds silicone particles or interacts with the immune system, making saline implants suspect as well.

Says Monona Rossol, an industrial hygienist and chemist specializing in silicones, "You have fluid moving in and around all the cells. A small molecule will float in the fluid and get into the lymph glands, the bloodstream, and migrate into tissues. You just don't know where the molecules are going to go." She likens this process to putting a toxic chemical underground. The water table, the direction the water is flowing, the rocky areas, and the streams—"compare [these] with blood, bone, tissue in people. The water is going to plume and move in its own way: it's difficult to predict what it's going to do."

Silicone can migrate another way as well. There is evidence that the body's protective enzymes break down the implant's silicone envelope; then immune-system cells called macrophages engulf the silicone particles. The macrophages carry the toxic silicone throughout the body, and in response the body releases immune chemicals called *cytokines*. These include interferon and tumor necrosis factor, which could be responsible for causing the flulike symptoms and other inflammatory symptoms, such as muscle pain and joint pain, suffered by some women with implants.

Rossol admits that immune problems in women with gel implants may be just a coincidence. On the other hand, she says, "It's absolutely outrageous that no one has studied this stuff. I can't believe the absolute arrogance of the medical profession and of Dow Chemical. How can they say the implants are safe when they don't know how much [silicone] stays in the implant, how much migrates, where it goes, or what it does in the body?"

The fact that silicone is widely used in medicine is often touted as proof of its safety. It is used to lubricate hypodermic needles for blood tests, to coat pacemakers, and in artificial joints. As Dr. Paul Striker asks, "If exposure to silicone is related to autoimmune disease, why don't we see more cases? Silicone has not been associated with problems in any other of its myriad uses. A juvenile-onset diabetic who administers a lifetime of insulin injections gets about the same amount of silicone as is contained in a gel implant—and if an implant ruptures, you don't even lose it all."

Rossol counters this observation. "How can they point to other silicone implants such as hip replacements as proof of safety when they don't know much about the recipients of these devices either? Where is the registry of these people? Where are the epidemiological studies of these recipients for symptoms of allergy or other diseases that may be related to silicone? It seems this industry mistakes lack of information and silence for endorsement of their product." Indeed, as Spiera points out, "Diabetes patients develop a kind of contracture in the joints, a fibrosis. This has been attributed to the disease, but one could make an argument that the silicone is causing this."

The silicone used for breast implants was not regulated, and implants vary as to the contaminants they contain. Because the implant manufacturers considered this to be proprietary information, we have no idea exactly what chemicals and contaminants the various implants made over the last four decades contain. Manufacturers have acknowledged that impurities are present, but no one has identified them all, nor do we have data about their biological effects in humans. According to Puzskin, there are at least thirty-seven substances in implants besides silicone, including benzene, formaldehyde, polyvinyl chloride, and printing ink.

A particularly troublesome class of chemicals is heavy metals, and it is one that Kolb is very concerned about because her patients often test positive for platinum, arsenic, and aluminum. The implants themselves may not contain the heavy metals, which are toxic to the body. Rather, the poisoning may be a "secondary" effect that is indirectly related to implants. Kolb says, "It might be that the implants are causing the liver to detox improperly, so the small amounts of these metals we are exposed to in normal life accumulate." The exception is platinum, which would almost certainly come from the implants, because very few people are exposed to platinum. (Platinum was commonly used as a catalyst in producing silicone.) Platinum in the body could also explain why so many women

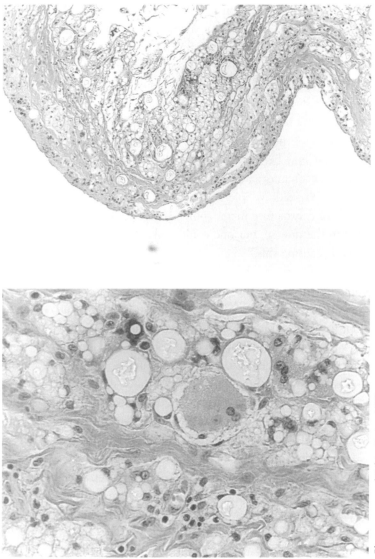

*These photographs, according to pathologist Rahim Karjoo, show that silicone from breast implants bleeds into surrounding tissue.* **Top:** *The clear portion (at the bottom of the photo) is a silicone implant; the top portion is the scar capsule with silicone bleed (small, clear, round shapes).* **Bottom:** *Silicone "lakes" (the clear portions) with gel crystals within them; the large opaque object in the center is a granuloma (a lump of chronically inflamed tissue).*

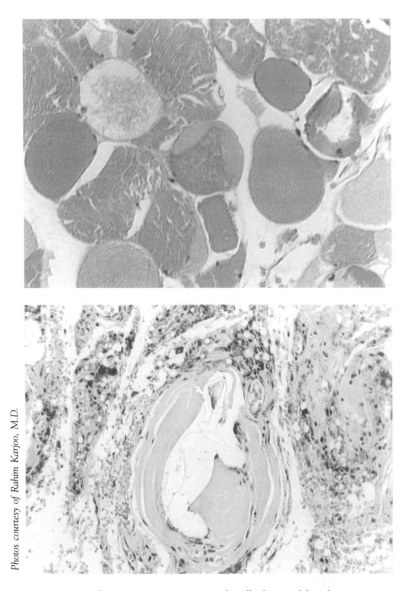

*Photos courtesy of Rahim Karjoo, M.D.*

**Top:** *The opaque masses are muscle cells destroyed by silicone.*
**Bottom:** *Breast tissue surrounding silicone (clear portion), which has polyurethane within it (the triangular shape).*

with implants develop lipomas (tumors consisting of fat cells), since platinum is associated with lipomas, according to Dr. Kolb.

## A Spectrum of Symptoms and Opinions

What this means for any individual woman, however, remains to be seen. The rheumatoid-like autoimmune diseases mentioned earlier are one possibility. But this theory is falling out of favor. The illness does not perfectly fit the criteria of this type of disease, so others have dubbed the disease "atypical" autoimmune disease or connective-tissue disease. The systemic symptoms that have been found in women with breast implants include weakness, chronic fatigue, muscle aches and pain (myalgia), joint pain and swelling, morning stiffness, memory problems, numbness, headache, Sjögren's-like syndrome (dry mouth, eyes, and vagina), vision problems, tingling, sweats, loss of balance, shortness of breath, gastrointestinal symptoms, bladder problems, swollen lymph nodes (lymphadenopathy), mysterious burning or crawling sensations, hair loss, fever, skin rashes, sore throats, allergies, dizziness, low-grade fevers, nausea, palpitations and chest pains that mimic heart attack, depression, and decreased sex drive.

Although these symptoms are remarkably diverse, they are also remarkably consistent. Dr. Arthur Brawer, an arthritis specialist and director of rheumatology at Monmouth Medical Center in New Jersey, writes, "[T]he term 'atypical' was very unfortunate, since we now know that silicone-induced disease is very typical for the patient who develops it." Proponents of the illness, he continues, know the "monotonous, repetitive, and redundant presentation of identical skin rashes and other multiple phenomena following implantation."

The spectrum of opinions is as broad as the spectrum of symptoms, and equally predictable. At one end are the skeptics: a large but slowly shrinking number of scientists and physicians (including most of the plastic surgeons who have been inserting implants for over thirty years) who generally believe this is much ado about nothing. They admit that a few women have local reactions such as breast hardening and implant rupture, and a few may suffer local granulomas (lumps) and inflammation, but that's all. At the other end are the "true believers," as rheumatologist Spiera calls them: a small but growing number of rheumatologists, immunologists, and plastic surgeons who are evaluating and treating thousands of women with symptoms, and pathologists who have microscopically examined implants and surrounding tissue. Some of them strongly feel there's no guarantee that anyone with any kind of breast implant is safe; they assert that no one should have silicone-gel breast implants or saline implants—or implants of any kind containing any form of silicone.

In the middle are those who feel that something is going on, but are not sure what. Some believe that, in women who are genetically predisposed to autoimmune disease, silicone may cause the disease to occur sooner or more severely. Some feel that certain women may be sensitive to silicone and suffer systemic immune problems even if they are not predisposed to autoimmune disease. But they believe the percentage of women who are vulnerable to silicone disease is very small, if it exists at all.

Melvin Spira, professor of surgery in the Division of Plastic Surgery and former head of plastic surgery at the Baylor College of Medicine, speaks for many plastic surgeons and other scientists when he says, "Every scientific study that has come out to date relative to implicating the silicone-gel implants with either autoimmune disease or connective-tissue disease has failed to do so. They have shown there is no cause and effect in scientific research that has been carried out by some very reputable researchers and published in high-quality peer-reviewed journals." He says he does not believe what he hears in the general media. "I feel very strongly that with possibly few exceptions, the over two million women that have been implanted have generally done well."

The believers—including the clinicians who have been treating the mysteriously ill women—say that nonbelievers are in denial or are living sheltered lives because sick women go for treatment to doctors other than their plastic surgeons, and because they are ignoring or misreading the studies that have been done so far.

## What Do the Studies Say?

Skeptics of systemic silicone disease point to a widely touted Mayo Clinic study published in *The New England Journal of Medicine* on 16 June 1994. In this study, the authors were unable to find an association between implants and a number of autoimmune diseases, including rheumatoid arthritis, systemic scleroderma, and systemic lupus. While hailed by some as the first major, published epidemiological study to evaluate silicone implants and autoimmune disorders, and to reassure women with implants, others point out that the study was faulty on several counts.

Instead of being based on doctors' exams of patients, it was based on nurses' reviews of the medical records of women with and without implants. Too few women were studied over too short a period of time. These diseases are relatively rare and have long latency periods, yet the 1994 study looked at only 749 women with implants and included women who'd received their implants as recently as 1991. The Mayo researchers themselves admitted it would require a sample of 62,000 women with implants and 124,000 women without implants, followed for an average of ten years each, to detect a doubling of the risk of scleroderma. And, as *Glamour* magazine pointed out the following September, "Not once in this detailed six-page article…do the researchers dare to make the statement 'Breast implants are safe.'" The author of the *Glamour* article, Amy Pagnozzi, also points out that in 1973 the Mayo Clinic claimed that daughters of women who took the morning-sickness drug DES did not have an increased risk of vaginal cancer. As we now know, this is untrue; the DES study had the same flaws as the silicone-implant study.

In addition, the study looked only for standard symptoms that define the classic form of these diseases, but silicone seems to be associated with symptoms that don't fit the mold. Monona Rossol says we are beginning to understand that the immune system mediates more than just the classic allergies. Silicone, she says, is not toxic in the classic sense. "If immune-mediated diseases can be triggered by nontoxic substances like plant pollen, some diseases might be triggered by silicone also. We're talking [about] an area where nobody has all the answers. The immune system is very complex."

Edward Knowlton, chief of plastic surgery at John Muir Hospital, says, "What the Mayo Clinic study doesn't show is whether silicone could act as an adjuvant [immune stimulant]. I think there is a relationship—although I think it's small—in patients who have a predilection for those diseases. There is a cause and effect as far as making these conditions worse in patients who are very likely to have them occur anyway." He emphasizes that "this risk does not exist in patients who don't have a predilection, and that's by far and away the majority of patients." He points out that any foreign body could conceivably act as an adjuvant: suture material (natural silk is far more reactive than synthetic sutures, interestingly), stainless steel in a hip implant, or the mesh (made of a plastic called Marlex) commonly used to replace fascia (such as during hernia repairs and for reinforcing the abdomen for a TRAM flap). "These are all much more bioreactive than the silicone envelope of a breast implant," according to Knowlton. "The reason that implants are made out of silicone in the first place is because it's the least bioreactive material we have."

The Mayo Clinic study is just one of seventeen epidemiological studies of autoimmune disease that were reviewed by the IOM. But these studies as a group are deeply flawed (see sidebar on the next page). This is the true meaning of junk science, and at least some government scientists recognize it as such.

Many studies have now been done on the scar capsule that surrounds the implant as to the amount of silicone in the capsular tissue and changes in the surrounding tissue. What they have found not only proves that silicone (gel and elastomer) enters the scar capsule, but that there is at least a local immune reaction to the implant. For example, a 1995 study by Canadian researchers compared the breast tissue of patients undergoing breast reduction with the fibrous capsules of patients with various types of implants. When compared with the tissue that had not been exposed to implants, they found that the capsules of women with silicone-gel

## FLAWED STUDIES

Many people think that just because a number of epidemiological studies cleared implants of classic autoimmune disease that implants are safe. Although the studies do show that most women don't develop classic autoimmune diseases after having implants for a short period of time, "any conclusions about the long-term safety of implants in terms of systemic disease are premature," says Dr. Diana Zuckerman. She points out that's because the studies, which were funded by implant manufacturers, have the following limitations:

◆ They used medical records and self-reports rather than clinical exams. One highly touted study (the Harvard Nurses' Study) included reports of women who claimed to have had implants since the 1950s—ten years before implants were invented;

◆ They focussed on classically defined autoimmune diseases and did not study most other diseases or atypical types of autoimmune disease;

◆ Most studies were too small to meaningfully study increases in the rare diseases they were studying;

◆ Most of the women studied had had their implants for too short a time—a few months or years—to develop the diseases that were the main focus of the studies. The Harvard Nurses' Study included women who'd had implants for only one month. We need to follow women for at least ten to fifteen years to reveal these diseases;

◆ Several of the studies were not even published in peer-reviewed journals—they were presented at scientific meetings or were written as doctoral dissertations.

breast implants had 108,000 times more silicone, men with silicone penis implants had 210 times more silicone, and women with saline implants had 83 times more silicone. In a 1997 study from Germany, the authors state that in at least 8.3 percent of the capsules they examined, they found signs of a local immune response. A study published in 1994 by a researcher from the Baylor University in Texas found not just scar capsules, but a cellular membrane resembling the synovium that normally lines the joints of the body. The smooth-surfaced implants had smooth membranes, but the textured ones had membranes that varied in thickness, and the inside surface of the membrane was "festooned with small (.25 to .5 mm) knob-like projections." He also found a "variety of foreign materials" either "within or adjacent to the capsules [which] included droplets of liquid silicone, irregular solid fragments of the bag envelope, geometric crystalline fragments of polyurethane, and talc.

Dr. Zuckerman says the poor quality of these studies is

> why I keep saying we don't know whether implants are safe over the long term, because the studies were not well enough designed to be persuasive. The information the IOM panel studied was based on studies that had substantial flaws. There was no federally funded research until recently. Virtually all research done was paid for by the manufacturers or plastic surgeons, and, not surprisingly, their research found that implants were safe. If the only research on cancer and smoking we had was funded by Phillip Morris, we would still be listening to their scientists who were saying there's an association but that doesn't mean causation.

Sure enough, shortly after the IOM panel wrote its report, three federally funded studies were published that raise serious questions about the long-term safety of implants. The studies were published in May 2001, and all found statistically significant increased health risks in women with implants. One of them, conducted by the FDA, was the first study ever to systematically follow women with ruptured implants. The researchers found that women with ruptured implants where the silicone gel had migrated out of the scar capsule were significantly more likely to report having fibromyalgia and several other painful and potentially fatal autoimmune diseases or related illnesses, such as dermatomyositis, polymyositis, Hashimoto's thyroiditis, pulmonary fibrosis, and polymyalgia.

The two other studies were conducted and funded by the National Cancer Institute. One of these found that when compared with women who'd undergone other forms of plastic surgery, women with implants were three times more likely to die of lung cancer, emphysema, and pneumonia. They were twice as likely to die from brain cancer. And they were four times more likely to commit suicide. The other NCI study found that, compared with other women of the same age, women with implants experienced a 21 percent increased risk of cancer overall—mainly brain cancer, respiratory-tract cancer, cervical cancer, leukemia, and vulvar cancer—and the number of certain cancers was twice as high. The lung–disease connection should not have been surprising, because the FDA study showed that women with ruptured breast implants had an increased likelihood of fibrosis of the lungs. Furthermore, the other NCI study of women with implants showed increased incidence of fatal lung disease. Interestingly, we also have evidence that silicone gel can migrate to the lungs; a woman with a calf implant began coughing up silicone of the same type found in her ruptured implant. If silicone could travel from the calf to the lung, how much easier for silicone from a breast implant to find its way to the much nearer lungs.

Another study found that in women who had rheumatological symptoms and silicone-gel-filled implants, 97 percent improved after their implants were removed. However, in 96 percent of the women who did not remove their implants, symptoms worsened.

Rheumatologist Harry Spiera was one of the first to notice a possible connection between silicone implants and connective-tissue disease. He has published papers about his own cases as well as a 1994 overview of other reported cases. By October 1994 he had seen seventeen patients with scleroderma: two had chin implants; the rest had silicone-gel breast implants. He says, "I'm convinced there is a relationship, but I couldn't convince a hostile audience." He points out that even if implants increase the frequency of scleroderma three times over (which is what Japanese researchers who studied silicone injections conclude), scleroderma is so rare that the numbers would still be quite small. And the concurrent development of disease in some women could be due to chance alone. The most generous published figures estimate that less than 0.03 percent of the general population has scleroderma. If 2,000,000 women have implants, that would mean 600 would have scleroderma by chance alone (2,000,000 times 0.0003). Rheumatoid arthritis has an estimated prevalence in the general population of 1–2 percent, so 20,000 to 40,000 women with implants would have it by chance. Fibromyalgia occurs in 7 percent of the general population, so 140,000 women with implants could be expected to have this condition. Their conditions could have nothing to do with implants—or the implants could, at the very least, make their symptoms come on sooner or with greater severity.

Frank Vasey is another rheumatologist who was among the first to suspect a link between silicone implants and autoimmune and rheumatic disorders. In his book *The Silicone Breast Implant Controversy*, he makes the case that we may be seeing a new disease. Dr. Vasey has treated over five hundred symptomatic women with silicone-gel implants. He explains that their symptoms differ from classic rheumatic conditions in that they experience "frequent muscle pain and tenderness in the anterior chest wall around the prosthesis and commonly describe an unusual burning character to the pain." He writes that under normal conditions, inflammation is a component of the healing process, but local inflammation provoked by silicone, if chronic, could create systemic effects and spread throughout the body.

Several groups of researchers have tested the blood and tissue of women with implants. Scientists debate the significance of these data, but they lend support to the notion of silicone-related immune disease that differs from other known immune disorders. For example, researchers have found evidence that both ruptured and intact implants cause inflammation, just as silicone injections do; this finding is a crucial factor in implicating the devices as a possible cause of immune disease. In 1993 Dow Corning revealed that new studies on laboratory rats showed that silicone gel used in implants was a strong irritant of the immune system. (This reinforces findings by 1974 Dow Chemical studies that the company failed to disclose to the FDA. The 1974 studies were revealed in a lawsuit.)

One-third of symptomatic patients with silicone breast implants have abnormal laboratory tests. For example, Nachman Brautbar and colleagues at the University of Southern California School of Medicine found that in the 40 women they studied, 28 percent had abnormal lymphocyte levels and 65 percent had elevated rheumatoid factor and immune complexes. Researchers have also found antibodies (substances the body produces to attack foreign substances such as viruses and bacteria) to silicone. In 1992 Randall Goldblum, at the University of Texas Medical Branch in Galveston, was the first to identify silicone antibodies; he found them in the blood of two children who had had silicone-coated tubes implanted to treat birth defects. In 1993 Suzanne Teuber and Eric Gershwin, at the University of California at Davis, found that among 100 women with implants, 35 had formed antibodies against their own collagen, a component of the connective tissue. By the end of 1994, Aristo Vojdani (Department of Medicine, Drew University School of Medicine and Science), Nachman Brautbar, and Alan Campbell (University of California School of Medicine) had published the results of their study of 520 symptomatic women with implants, in whom they found antibodies to silicone.

Britta Ostermeyer Shoaib and Bernard M. Patten, of the Baylor College of Medicine, studied 1,500 women who developed autoimmune disease after breast-implant surgery. Many of them had signs of neurological as well as rheumatological disease. The patients usually had abnormal blood tests and other abnormal tissue tests, such as immunoglobulins, auto-antibodies, and degenerating and atrophied nerves in the biceps and pectoralis muscles. In one report, 12 women had developed a multiple sclerosis–like syndrome. Among the first 100 women they evaluated, 81 reported memory problems; when they tested 15 of those women, brain scans showed statistically significant changes, and memory tests showed lower than average performance in several areas. Because of their experiences with these patients, the researchers believe silicone may damage the nervous system indirectly by autoimmune mechanisms.

Many women do complain of cognitive problems—brain fog, memory loss, confusion—and many of them are in their twenties and thirties, so their problems cannot be shrugged off as just part of getting older. Positron-emission tomography (PET) scans have shown that women with implants have brain abnormalities, and that these decrease when they have their implants removed. Other studies show that women with silicone-gel breast implants have a high incidence of electroencephalogram (EEG) abnormalities.

Women with symptoms that may be due to their implants have a wide range of reactions:

◆ I know my constellation of symptoms could develop anytime, in anyone. But no one else in my family has any of them. I have dry eye, and was prone to a lot of infections and problems and misdiagnosed by several doctors before we figured out what it was. I have a dry mouth, which may be linked to my gum problems. I've had a series of respiratory infections, and a strange chronic irritation in my nasal passages. I have an ache in my foot, in one joint in my toe, that becomes sharp at times—I'm concerned because I walk a lot and jog. I have mild rheumatoid-like symptoms in my hands, which ache, and I have poor circulation. I have degenerative connective tissue in my eyes—this happens to older people [this woman was in her early forties when interviewed]. My memory loss I attribute to the anesthesia. I'm still not sure there's a connection, but when I saw the list of silicone-associated symptoms, something clicked.

◆ After my fourth implant to replace the one that had contracted, I woke up from the surgery with my right hand stiff and sore. I couldn't bend my fingers. My plastic surgeon told me later that my implant had ruptured and he had to flush out the silicone with saline. Soon after, the FDA hearings put the issue all over the front pages of the newspapers. I thought there might be a connection, but when I told him about the pain in my hand, he said it was pure coincidence—did arthritis run in my family? But I only had one aunt with rheumatoid arthritis. I now have an allergy to yeast, mold, and fungus. Except for the cancer, I've always been healthy, never any allergies. I'm tired and weak. I have dry eyes and a dry vagina. I wake up with my eyes stuck together. I've suddenly developed visual problems, huge floaters. I'm convinced my problems are due to silicone. I can't buy that my hand problems would just suddenly be triggered by an operation—that it was in my genes just waiting to happen.

◆　I've talked to many other women with implants and most of them have...neurological problems with their hands and arms. Their muscles are weak just like mine—I can't lift and move things that ordinarily I could do with ease. I strain my muscles easily and have pain for months. I forget things easily, miss appointments, can't do or remember more than one thing at a time. I suppose you could blame some of these symptoms on menopause, but my sister is two years older than me and she doesn't have arthritic hands, or dry eyes, or weakness, or muscle cramps. She's still energetic and I'm not. I had silicone injections first, then I had silicone implants to replace the breast tissue that was surgically removed because of lumps and calcium deposits. Silicone has also formed lumps under my arms, in my thyroid, back, and female organs, and I've had my thyroid removed. I've got bad headaches. I've had half my teeth removed because the silicone caused abscesses; now I'm having trouble with my partial because I've got dry mouth. Silicone has migrated to my optic nerve and I go blind for one and a half hours at a time.

I used to be an accountant; I used to have total recall. I could tell you the type of wallpaper I had in my room as a child, what people wore—not anymore. There are days I can't even keep up a conversation on the phone. My sister has had implants for seventeen years and doesn't have any symptoms. But she has suddenly developed a lot of allergies—could they be related to silicone? I think a lot of women are in denial. How many have symptoms and don't recognize they could be related to silicone? I was diagnosed with the flu and it was really chronic fatigue. One doctor said my lumpy breasts were due to cola, coffee, and cigarettes! It's mind-boggling when you get into it—we have to laugh at ourselves, some of the stories are so insane. I've been told that we're a unique group—because we're still alive.

## The Role of Infection

An interesting theory is that, in some cases, many of the symptoms blamed on silicone could be due to a systemic bacterial or fungal infection. Richard V. Dowden wrote an article published in 1994 proposing this theory, based on a small study of seven women. The women all experienced systemic symptoms including malaise, fatigue (sometimes debilitating), muscle aches, joint pain, insomnia, diarrhea, irregular menstrual periods, and memory impairment; most also suffered from capsular contracture (severe in three of the women), local pain, and discomfort.

Dr. Dowden removed their implants and found that only one implant had ruptured, and one had a "pinpoint leak"; one woman had a single saline implant. He observed that the systemic symptoms rapidly resolved in all seven patients after they received an antibacterial regimen and had their implants removed. In five patients, he was able to culture two types of bacteria from around the implants: *Staphylococcus epidermidis* and *Propionibacterium acnes*. He writes that although these bacteria are very common and usually harmless, the women may have experienced an "idiosyncratic response" to them.

Dowden also writes, "[W]hen symptoms abate after implant removal, there is a temptation to jump to the conclusion that the cause was silicone." However, he feels low-virulence bacteria could be the cause, for several reasons. First, he left the scar capsule (presumably containing silicone molecules) in place; second, "virtually all adults in the U.S. are walking around with silicone in their bodies that cannot be removed." Yet, the women improved "dramatically, completely, and rapidly, despite the fact that silicone not only remained in their bodies but also had been present prior to insertion of the implants." Dowden also believes that "individual susceptibility plays a role" in the likelihood that the common bacteria would cause a problem in a particular woman. He estimates that, based on his own statistics and discussion with other plastic surgeons, one in one thousand implant patients are susceptible to developing these symptoms.

Edward Knowlton believes Dowden's theory has merit. He says he has had patients who get implants and "afterward, they just don't feel good, and they may be feeling rotten due to the organism." He adds:

> There are a number of studies that show that when a foreign body is added to the body, the number of bacteria needed to cause an infection is greatly reduced. *S. epidermidis*…is beneficial, it protects us like a shield against other harmful bacteria such as strep. Women who don't have *S. epidermidis* in their breasts may tend to get breast abscesses. But when a foreign body such as many sutures or an implant is also present, you can get a constant indolent infection which in many women with breast implants is expressed as capsular contraction, or in certain patients as these flulike symptoms—and that may be a lot of patients.

Dr. Susan Kolb feels infection is a factor in her patients' illnesses, especially if they have textured implants. She has found that when she removes silicone-gel implants, about half contain pathogenic organisms such as *Staph aureus* and enterococcus, and 95 percent of the saline implants test positive. She has removed several saline implants that were black with what she believes was fungus—fungus that could migrate into the bloodstream and cause many of the symptoms associated with implants. Many of her patients have been told by their plastic surgeons or their rheumatologists that their implants are not making them sick, only to discover abnormal bacterial and fungal growth around an implant. When the implant is removed, and the patients are properly treated, which she says includes antibiotics and antifungal treatment as appropriate, they recover and their health improves.

Dr. Kolb also believes there is "another newly emerging disease with saline implants that is different than the one with silicone gel." Her theory is that textured implants—most of which are saline-filled—not only get more readily infected than do smooth implants, but that a certain foam used in the formation of the textured surface may not be completely removed, exposure to which causes a multiple chemical sensitivity.

## A Continuum of Symptoms?

Dr. Susan Kolb theorizes, "The first element of silicone disease has to do with the development of systemic candidiasis due to an immune dysfunction which I have found to be associated with depressed natural killer T-cell levels." She proposes:

> Once the silicone gel leaks out of the implant, a chronic immune response occurs that is often associated with local capsular bacterial infection and with systemic and possibly local fungal infections. The patients next experience neurological problems that can be explained by the silicone gel migrating directly or via the macrophages into the lymphatic and nervous systems. Women with longstanding silicone-gel exposure have typical neurological problems, usually beginning in the extremity on the side of the implant that leaks or ruptures first. Some women [also] have toxicity from platinum and other chemicals that are used in the manufacturing process of the implants. In my experience, the end stage of this disease is an autoimmune condition similar to scleroderma. It may be modulated by intracellular bacterial infections that change the characteristics of the cell wall and lead to autoimmune symptoms that are atypical. This does not occur right away and may take ten or more years of silicone exposure.

Nancy Carteron, a rheumatologist, has seen hundreds of women with symptoms. She believes it is best to look at the potential harms as existing on a continuum, with most people still at the beginning stages of the process. She summarizes what she has concluded, based on her hands-on evaluation and the handful of studies done so far:

◆ **Women with no problems yet:** Some people with implants have had no problems whatsoever, although there clearly is a direct correlation between the length of time the implants are in and either leakage or rupture and resulting local problems.

◆ **Women with local problems:** The next group is people with capsular contracture, pain, hardening, and decreased sensation in breast and nipple. But the difficulties are still limited to the chest wall and breast area.

◆ **The transition from local to regional:** It seems a smaller subset of people begin to get a neurological-type pain that spreads from the chest wall up into the neck and shoulder area. Often—but not always—this is later correlated with the side on which an implant ruptured.

◆ **Women with systemic problems:** After the pain spreads within the immediate area, people seem to then develop a lot of systemic symptoms. These can range from just a few pains throughout the body—muscle and joint aches—to arthralgia, painful joints that wax and wane without actual joint inflammation. There can be lymph-node swelling, low-grade fever, and rashes that are often local to chest or arms but can occur anywhere.

Dr. Carteron believes that although it may be easier for people to understand local and systemic symptoms as separate entities, it is more appropriate to think of them as a continuum. "They're not home free if they've just got local symptoms right now," she warns. "Symptoms seem to follow one after the other, and if you go back and look at the history of people who have systemic symptoms, you see the pattern."

Brautbar, Vasey, and others present as further evidence for cause and effect that, according to various reports, 50 to 70 percent of patients who developed symptoms following implantation recovered or improved after their implants were removed. This improvement is usually gradual, sometimes beginning up to twelve months after explantation, supporting the notion that the improvement was not due to the placebo effect, which generally occurs immediately. Removal of the implants and the scar capsule reduces the amount of silicone in the body, and the delayed gradual improvement suggests that the decrease in silicone has allowed normal immune function to reassert itself. Even if the explantation ignores silicone that has migrated to other parts of the body, the amount left behind may be too small to stimulate an abnormal immune response. However, in some women, the remaining silicone may be enough to maintain the immune disorder, and this could be one explanation as to why some women do not improve after their implants are removed.

## Immune or Autoimmune?

In October 1994, Dr. David Smalley and colleagues at the University of Tennessee presented what appears to be compelling evidence of a direct cause and effect: Silicone can cause immune disease. Their report involves a woman who had received implants in 1973 and developed rheumatic symptoms. She had her implants removed, and after fourteen months almost all her symptoms improved. Two and a half years after explantation, Dr. Smalley tested her immune system and found that it was only slightly sensitive to silicon dioxide (a component of the elastomer shell). Soon after, the woman underwent surgery to remove her scar capsule; it was found to be full of silica, and as a result of the surgery she was re-exposed to silica from her implants. Her symptoms rapidly reappeared, and immunologic testing three weeks after surgery revealed that her immune system reacted to silica eight times more strongly than normal; eight weeks after surgery it was twelve times the normal level. Six months postsurgery, however, her immune system response had returned to normal. Smalley believes this is the first case ever to prove that silicone from breast implants can be a direct cause of immune problems. "Clearly," he says, "when we took away the stimulant the immune system quieted down." Smalley, who since the 1980s has concentrated on clinical immunology, recently specialized in cell-mediated immune response to silicone and silica as it relates to clinical disease. His work supporting a silicone–immune disease link includes a study showing that symptomatic silicone-implant recipients do respond immunologically to silicon dioxide, when compared with normal patients and people with rheumatoid disease but no implants.

However, the jury is still out on this one, and it may be that in some women it is autoimmune and in others it is not. Carteron stresses the importance of understanding the distinction between an *autoimmune* response and an *immune* response. This distinction may provide one explanation for the inconsistency in recovery. An autoimmune response, once set in motion, is very difficult to turn off completely, she says. "You're making an antibody to something in your own tissue, so you never can get rid of that potential completely—you can down-regulate it, you can modulate it, you can put it into remission, but you can't get rid of the heart tissue or the joint-lining tissue that the antibodies are reacting to. Whereas if it's a reaction to a foreign substance [an immune response], if you got rid of the foreign substance, the detrimental cascade of symptoms should decrease." She continues:

> The focus when this controversy first developed was on true autoimmune diseases like scleroderma and lupus. Historically there were reasons to be concerned about that. From the Japanese data on injected silicone, there does appear to be an association between silicone and a development of these diseases. But most of the epidemiological studies that are available to date [such as the Mayo Clinic study mentioned earlier in this chapter] say that there is probably no association or minimal association with typical autoimmune disease. I think there's a potential to develop an autoimmune process from silicone, but the incidence has to be really low;...what the numbers are and the risk factors [such as genetic predisposition] are we don't know yet.

Carteron feels that people with symptoms do not have a bona fide autoimmune disorder. "It appears to be an immune reaction to a foreign substance, but they haven't developed a true auto-antibody response." If true, this is good news, because it gives them a better chance for recovery.

David Borenstein, professor of medicine at the Division of Rheumatology at George Washington University, points out that the major symptoms—overwhelming fatigue, joint and muscle pain—are reminiscent of a flulike state. He proposes that a likely source for these constitutional symptoms are the substances released by the immune system (antibodies and cytokines) during viral infection and when immune cells digest silicone molecules. Researchers have found a number of immunologically active factors around intact implants, and studies suggest that some people are genetically predisposed toward chronic inflammation and production of these factors.

Borenstein concludes by saying, "The current controversy involving silicone breast implants seems reminiscent of the debate surrounding the original patients with Lyme disease." Early patients were children with arthritislike symptoms, and they were diagnosed with juvenile rheumatoid arthritis. However, we eventually discovered that adults were also affected and that what we were really seeing was a new disease transmitted by a tick. Although the mechanism is not yet clear, what we are seeing with breast implants seems to be a new disease "transmitted" by silicone.

## Are You Feeling Lucky?

Will everyone with implants eventually have a reaction to silicone? "That's a tough question," admits Nancy Carteron, the rheumatologist who proposes viewing symptoms on a continuum. Whether you experience symptoms may be a matter of time and individual chemistry. But she does have some thoughts:

> I was an immunologist and a virologist before I practiced rheumatology, and I think it will turn out to be multifactorial. There will be some people that may have a genetic predisposition to developing a reaction, or may develop it

earlier. But I think that the risk for it clearly would increase with time, because it seems that these things [implants] don't last very long in the human body. The higher the quantity of exposure, the more likely it is that one would react.

Time, then, is a factor because of wear and tear on the implant and duration of exposure. Individual chemistry is a factor because of predisposition and strength of immune reaction. Carteron continues:

> I don't think everyone will develop it, no matter how long it's been implanted. But there's no way to know who would or who wouldn't, or whether that will be what the finding is. However, quite clearly in human breast tissue there is a reaction to the substance, and it seems like a foreign-body reaction. It would seem highly likely that this would occur in a large number of people.... There's a lot of speculation, but not a lot of data to stand on. They've been around long enough that maybe after the data are collated from the evaluations for the purposes of the settlement, there will be a little bit better information.

Dowden asserts that the ramifications of this theory go far beyond breast implants. He feels it is probable that a percentage of all implanted devices may trigger similar symptoms. Women with breast implants tend to be younger (and generally healthier) than other implant patients. In people with hip replacements or pacemakers, for example, symptoms such as fatigue and aches and pains may be blamed on the person's age or underlying disorder, rather than on the implant.

## Cancer

There has been concern that women with breast implants may be at higher risk of breast cancer and other types of cancers, that implants might delay the detection of breast cancer, and that implants might increase the risk of cancer recurrence or decrease the length of survival after a diagnosis of breast cancer.

## Breast Cancer

Although breast implants may interfere with the diagnosis of breast cancer (see the section in Chapter 4 titled "Interference with Mammography and Cancer Detection"), there is no evidence that implants cause breast cancer. In 2000, NCI researchers published the results of a reassuring study of 13,500 women who had breast implants for augmentation. They compared them with two other groups: women in the general population, and 4,000 women who had other forms of plastic surgery. This was because augmentation patients and women who get other forms of plastic surgery share common risk factors for breast cancer, so the researchers thought this might have been a more appropriate comparison group than women in general. This study was not only large; it was long term: They followed the women for an average of thirteen years. What they found was that "there was no change in breast cancer risk," according to Louise Brinton, the principle investigator in the study. However, they did find that breast cancer was detected at a somewhat later stage in the implant patients, but that this difference was not statistically significant and there was no significant difference in death rates between the implant and comparison groups.

This study supports the results of two other large-scale studies that were published in 1992. A Canadian study by Hans Berkel (Alberta Cancer Board in Edmonton) and colleagues compared 11,676 women who had breast augmentation from 1973 through 1986 with 13,557 women without implants. Forty-one patients with implants were found to have breast cancer, versus the expected figure of 86.2.

The other study, by Dennis Deapan and Garry Brody, at the University of Southern California School of Medicine, is even more reassuring. It involved 3,112 Los Angeles County women who reported receiving implants for breast augmentation from 1959 to 1980, with 91 percent in the years 1970 to 1980. Twenty-one of the women with breast implants were diagnosed with breast cancer—lower than the expected incidence of 31.7, based on Los

Angeles County incidence rates. Other cancers were similarly unexpectedly low: 45 incidences were diagnosed, but 50 were expected. The authors speculate that one reason for the markedly lower than average rate for breast cancer could be that women who are at higher risk for this disease (because of family history, for example) might be less likely to opt for augmentation out of the belief that implants "might further increase the risk or inhibit detection," putting the augmented women at slightly lower risk than the general population. Another theory is that women who have augmentation are at a lower risk because they have smaller breasts and less breast tissue, but there are no studies to support this hypothesis.

However, none of these studies included women who had implants for breast reconstruction after breast cancer. So we do not know what the effect of breast implants might be on these women, who are at risk for a recurrence of the original cancer, and who are also at higher than average risk for a second primary breast cancer in the other breast.

## Other Cancers

What about other cancers? When the FDA issued its 1993 report, the only studies that existed were those done with laboratory animals. We now have reliable human studies, conducted by the NCI. Two recent studies, conducted by researchers at NCI and mentioned earlier in this chapter, did find a link between breast implants and certain forms of cancer. One found that women who have breast implants are at a higher risk of dying from brain tumors and lung cancer (as well as from suicide). The other federally funded study found that women with implants have a 21 percent increase in the risk of getting cancer in general, compared with women of the same age without implants.

In polyurethane-coated implants there is the additional risk of the foam coating breaking down in the body. In the process, it releases a chemical called TDA (2-toluenediamine) that has been proven to cause liver cancer in rats and is suspected of being carcinogenic in humans. TDA was removed from hair dye in 1971 because of its carcinogenicity. In 1993, the results of a year-long study that examined sixty women with polyurethane-coated implants and sixty women without implants were released. The women with implants were found to have small amounts of TDA in their blood and urine; the women without implants had none. The amounts of the chemical were small—in the parts-per-trillion range—and the FDA said it was uncertain what the risk of cancer would be.

According to calculations released by the FDA, the cancer risk from polyurethane-coated implants, if any, is likely to be very small. They estimate the lifetime risk for a woman with two implants to be less than one in a million if she had implants for thirty-five years. Despite this opinion, in one lawsuit the jury found for the plaintiff, deciding that the foam was a contributing factor in the acceleration of a preexisting potential cancer in her breast. Because of this risk and other problems, including the presence of TDA in breast milk in women with these implants, the manufacturers took foam-coated implants off the market in 1991, but not before an estimated one hundred thousand women had received these implants. Any calculation of the risk of developing cancer from this type of implant needs to consider the fact that many women had more than one foam implant in each breast—either because the original implants were replaced or because surgeons sometimes "stacked" or doubled up implants in one breast—which would increase their exposure to this dangerous substance.

## Effects During Pregnancy and Breast-Feeding

Some scientists have raised the question of whether migrating silicone in a pregnant woman could have an adverse effect on her fetus, or on a baby who is being breast-fed by a mother with implants. Although the IOM report concludes that there is no evidence of harm, several studies have caused concern.

Suzanne S. Teuber, a rheumatologist at the University of California at Davis, reported in 1994 about two young children whose mothers had silicone-gel breast implants. Both children were breast-fed for about three months, and both had persistent diffuse aches and pains that caused them to complain as soon as they could talk. They also had elevated ANA (antinuclear antibody) levels, indicating a stimulation of the immune system. Teuber is concerned that "these two children may reflect a new clinical syndrome" and writes that "more research is needed to determine whether it is possible for silicone or silicone breakdown products from a ruptured or leaking implant to pass into breast milk or across the placenta. If this is possible, these substances may interact with a child's immune system."

Another report published in 1994 studied eleven children of mothers with silicone breast implants, eight of whom were breast-fed. Jeremiah Levine (Albert Einstein College of Medicine), the lead researcher, found that six of the breast-fed children had a stiffening of the esophagus, which makes swallowing difficult, but the other children did not. The researchers said, "It is unclear whether the silicone itself, other by-products released by the implants, or immunologic factors, such as immune cells or antibodies," may have contributed to the condition. "The possibility that they may develop scleroderma-like esophageal disease suggests that these children may constitute another group of patients at risk for developing disease related to exposure to breast implants." An accompanying editorial tempered these findings by reviewing the many benefits of breast-feeding, and mentions that advising against breast-feeding may not spare babies from exposure, since bottle nipples and pacifiers contain silicone.

David Smalley and colleagues at the University of Tennessee demonstrated that children of symptomatic women also have unusual symptoms, such as esophageal problems, arthralgia, growth

disorder, and abdominal pains; that they also respond immunologically to silicone; and that they therefore must have been exposed
to silicone via the placenta and possibly via breast milk.

Silicone implants covered with polyurethane foam may pose a
risk to nursing infants if the carcinogen TDA enters breast milk.
The FDA says they have one report that a trace amount of TDA
may have been found in one out of three samples of breast milk
from one woman. At this point, however, there is no conclusive
evidence that either fetuses or nursing infants could be harmed by
polyurethane-coated silicone implants.

# 6

# What Should You Do if You Have an Implant?

Because of the recent doubts about the safety of implants, the biggest questions facing women with implants are: What shape are my implants in? Are they ruptured, leaking, intact? If I am having symptoms, are they due to my implants? Should I have them removed? If so, how extensive does the surgery have to be? Should I have them replaced?

While we don't know how long any particular implant will last, we do know they all will fail at some point and need to be removed and, if the woman wishes, replaced—even if she doesn't notice any symptoms. The FDA believes there is not enough evidence to justify having intact silicone implants removed if you are not having symptoms. Most plastic surgeons, women's health groups, and consumer groups agree. However, since the average "body life" of an implant is estimated at eight to ten years, most women will probably need their implants replaced at least once in their lives. If you have implants when you are very young—say, in your twenties, you may have five or more surgeries ahead of you. Even in the absence of physical symptoms, peace of mind may be enough reason to consider implant removal. How can we know when they should be removed? And what can we do to safeguard our emotional and physical health and be on the alert for potential problems?

As is the case with the question of systemic disease, the medical community does not agree as to what circumstances justify that a woman have her implants removed, when she should be tested to see if the implants are ruptured or if the silicone has spread beyond the capsule, or how this testing should occur. They don't agree on whether the capsule should be removed along with the implants, and whether the tests available are a valid indication of an immune reaction to silicone.

## General Steps

Experts agree that the best course of action begins with the following general steps:

**Establish an ongoing relationship with your plastic surgeon, so you can discuss your concerns freely.** If your surgeon does not fill this need, or if you cannot remember or locate your original plastic surgeon, find another one you can speak frankly with. Edward Knowlton, chief of plastic surgery at John Muir Medical Center, feels strongly that plastic surgeons should spend time talking with their patients about the issues. "We're not totally blameless that patients went through the terror of watching a totally unscientific debate take place in the media, and that they now have to bear this extra burden of anxiety and doubt." A compassionate, understanding surgeon can go a long way in calming any undue fear you may have and steering you through the decisions ahead of you.

**Find out what kind of implant you have, the name of the manufacturer, the date it was implanted, and the model number.** You may need to do a bit of detective work, but this information should be part of your medical record. Contact your plastic surgeon or the facility where the implant surgery was performed. Some women have been told that they have saline implants, when they actually were given silicone implants. The type and year of your implants can offer clues as to their condition and what steps you should take, if any.

Once you know which implant you have, get the informational material (package insert) that comes with it and describes the possible adverse effects. When we first got our implants, many of us were not told everything we needed to know, or we neglected to ask. Most of us did not know to ask for—nor were we offered—the package insert, which contains a wealth of information, including a bibliography of pertinent scientific studies on the possible adverse effects. In calling the manufacturer (see the Resources section for toll-free phone numbers), you may find you must enlist the aid of your doctor, because some will send package inserts to physicians only, not directly to patients.

Be aware that the chance of an implant rupture increases the longer you have it; therefore, the older your implant, the more vigilant you must be in your self-monitoring and professional monitoring. Although there is no agreement on this issue, some believe the risk of rupture increases with physical stress on the implant. According to the manufacturer's literature, your risk of a ruptured or leaking implant may increase if your lifestyle imposes "excessive stresses or manipulation as may occur during normal living experiences including routine and purposeful trauma as in vigorous exercise, athletics, and intimate physical contact." Others warn that "Excessive manipulation of the implant shell during use" such as "routine manual massage or manual exercise of the implanted breast may also produce long-term fatigue of the envelope, resulting in rupture." While "excessive stress" and "excessive trauma" are difficult to define, most plastic surgeons feel it is unnecessary to curtail common forms of physical activity such as dance, calisthenics, weight lifting, jogging, and aerobic dance, even though they may be high impact and jar or rub the implant envelope. One woman told me that her surgeon warned her away from certain sexual positions. On the other hand, Richard Jobe, of Stanford University Medical Center, says, "It doesn't make any sense to me. The implants are designed to be highly elastic. I don't think the risk is sufficient to modify your behavior. I think the warning is just another way of transferring responsibility to the patient, of making her feel like she might be the reason for the problem if it develops." Still, you may feel more comfortable if you wear a good sports bra that gives you support and minimizes breast movement. And if you are physically active, you might want to be especially careful to avoid trauma to the breast, which might occur from falls or very active sports. Many women rupture their implants when they are in car accidents or during a fall in which their breasts are injured.

**Report any problems you are having with your implant to MedWatch, the FDA Medical Products Reporting Program.** For consumers, the phone number is (888) 463-6332. They will send you a form to fill out, or you may go to the web and download the report form at: www.fda.gov/medwatch/index.html. Although you must give them your name, your privacy will be protected. This is one way the FDA collects information about problems.

**You might also find it useful to talk to other women individually or in a support group, or to a therapist, or to use both to help you deal with emotional concerns you might have about your implants.** The groups listed in the Resources section will be able to provide psychological support over the phone and refer you to other individuals and groups in your area. Some women find support groups—including those proliferating on the web—to be an emotional oasis and a fund of information. But the nature and quality of support groups vary, and they are not for everyone. Some women complain that hearing the horror stories of group members provokes rather than calms their anxieties. You may need to search a bit for a group that is more supportive and less destructive.

## Guidelines for Self-Monitoring

Monitor your health, following the guidelines listed below, to help detect problems as early as possible. The earlier problems are recognized, the better your chance of obtaining successful treatment.

## Breast Self-Exam (BSE)

All women, implants or no, should examine their breasts once a month to detect changes that could mean breast cancer. If you have implants, you need to be especially vigilant because breast self-exams can also help detect ruptures. Ask your doctor to help you learn how to distinguish between your own breast tissue and your implant—it can be confusing at first. If you are still menstruating, the best time to perform the exam is two or three days after your period has ended, when your breasts are least likely to be tender or swollen.

To perform BSE, stand in front of a mirror and look for any unusual changes, such as dimples, lumps, or nipple discharge. Look first with both arms raised, and then lowered. Next, raise one arm at a time and feel for lumps or masses in the breast with the flat surface of the fingertips of the opposite hand. Also feel for lumps or swelling in the armpit. Then repeat the exam while lying down. The American Cancer Society, hospitals, and breast health centers offer booklets, videotapes, and training sessions with detailed instructions about breast self-exam.

During the exam, and as you go about your daily activities, watch for the following, which may be signs of a leak or rupture:

- ◆ tenderness, lumpiness, or discomfort around the implant
- ◆ change in the shape of your breast
- ◆ change in the consistency of your breast, such as increased softness
- ◆ change in the way your breast moves

Call your plastic surgeon if you suspect a rupture. If your implant has ruptured, most experts advise that you have it removed as soon as possible and have the gel cleaned out of the area.

## Other Possible Warning Signs

Be alert to any other signs and symptoms in other parts of your body. These include:

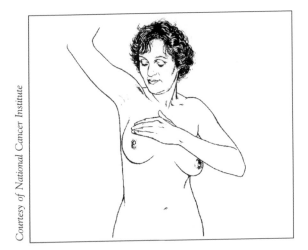

*Courtesy of National Cancer Institute*

*Self-monitoring for implant problems and breast cancer includes a monthly breast self-exam (BSE).*

◆ hardening of breast tissue

◆ muscle pain

◆ pain and swelling of the joints

◆ pain in the soft tissues

◆ a burning sensation of pain

◆ tightness, redness, or swelling of the skin

◆ swollen glands or lymph nodes

◆ unusual, extreme, or unexplained fatigue

◆ swelling of the hands and feet

◆ unusual hair loss

◆ rashes

◆ skin thickening or hardening

◆ dry eyes, mouth, or vagina

◆ loss of memory, or mental confusion and "fogginess"

◆ any of the other symptoms mentioned in Chapter 5

These could indicate a variety of health problems, some of which may be linked to implants. If you experience these symptoms, particularly more than one, and if they do not go away, see your doctor or plastic surgeon for an evaluation. He or she may refer you to another specialist, such as an internist, an allergist, or a rheumatologist.

## Guidelines for Professional Monitoring

You should also be watched professionally for signs of rupture or leakage. Saline-filled implants usually deflate rapidly after breaking, resulting in obvious changes. But ruptured or leaking silicone-gel implants do not always show obvious changes, such as alteration in size or shape. The FDA and the medical community therefore recommend that you have regular professional exams even if you are not experiencing symptoms related to implants. Because implants can interfere with mammograms and breast exams, these types of routine screenings are probably not adequate. You need to make sure you receive high-quality cancer screening.

### Regular Physical Exams

Make annual appointments with your plastic surgeon, gynecologist, internist, or nurse practitioner for a thorough examination, which may detect subtle changes in your breast that could indicate a leak or rupture, or other health problems related to your implant. Your doctor should take a thorough history and ask whether there is any breast cancer or autoimmune diseases in your family, including the age at diagnosis and the outcome of the disease; whether you have a history of breast lumps or treatments; other factors that might increase your risk of breast cancer; and your implant history, including date of implantation, complications, open or closed capsulectomy, and other incidents and symptoms.

It is usually more complicated and difficult to physically examine augmented breasts, but also more important because implants can obscure breast tissue on a mammogram, and the human touch may catch something the machine misses. Neal Handel feels that since plastic surgeons are the most knowledgeable about implants, they are your best choice for regular monitoring. Some surgeons claim they are able to do a "pinch test," in which they squeeze the implant; it is ruptured if it feels as though toothpaste is being squeezed out of a tube. Other physicians are less likely to be able to distinguish normal from abnormal features associated with implants. Implants have seams, folds, valves, and sealing patches that could easily mislead an inexperienced examiner. Likewise, bumps that might arouse suspicion in a practiced hand might be dismissed as implant features and wrongly ignored by a physician less familiar with implants.

In addition to a physical exam, you should have your breasts imaged to screen for breast cancer and to see:

◆ whether an implant is intact or ruptured

◆ if it has ruptured, whether it is fully or partially collapsed and whether the silicone is still contained in the scar capsule

◆ if silicone is found outside the capsule, how much has escaped and where it has migrated to

This information will help you decide whether you should remove your implants and, if the answer is yes, how extensive the surgery should be.

In one study, 204 women with implants were evaluated by MRI. Thirty-nine decided to have their implants removed. Of the 39, all had ruptured implants, but the surgeon, based on a physical exam, had predicted that only 4 would be ruptured. The rest were "silent" ruptures, undetected by physical exam and questioning, and which have a much better chance of being detected by MRI. MRI helped the surgeons develop the operative plan, including the number and location of the incisions and the way the surgeon approached the silicone outside the capsule, all of which presumably improved the outcome of the surgery.

When I decided to have my sixteen-year-old double-lumen implant removed in 1998, I consulted with my plastic surgeon as to whether I should have an MRI to see if it had ruptured. Rupture of the silicone envelope was likely, considering the implant's age and the fact that an earlier MRI had shown that the outer saline lumen had ruptured. She said, "Don't bother, I've never seen a ruptured implant of your type. And it won't change anything in the surgery." I regretted not having the MRI, because it would have shown that the implant had ruptured and would have prepared me for the more extensive surgery I needed as a result.

## Special Mammography

If you are in the age group for whom routine mammograms are recommended (age forty and up), realize that although low-cost, mass-screening mammography may be adequate for women without breast implants, if you have implants you will need more individualized and specialized attention. Tell the radiologist that you have implants so he or she can take special care to avoid rupturing the implant when compressing your breast.

Ask to see the facility's accreditation by the American College of Radiology; accredited facilities are more likely to have radiologists and technicians with the specialized training you need. Call the American Cancer Society's or the Cancer Information Service's toll-free line for a list of certified mammography centers in your area (see Resources).

Make every effort to visit a breast center that is experienced in taking and reading mammograms in women who have implants. In addition to the routine compression mammogram (top and side views), you may require additional views to image as much breast tissue as possible. (An implant prevents up to 50 percent—and possibly more—of the breast tissue from being seen on a mammogram. Even saline obscures low-density masses and most fine microcalcifications, as well as most high-density masses.) Try to find someone experienced in *displacement mammography* (also called the Eklund technique—after its originator—or the pinch technique), an alternative or addition to compression mammography. Most radiologists agree this method significantly improves the image quality and the amount of breast tissue imaged.

Since displacement allows the anterior (front) of the breast to be seen best, and compression reveals more posterior (rear) tissue, both methods together may show more breast than either one alone. In women with severe capsular contraction, however, displacement mammography shows less breast tissue than standard compression mammography. The situation varies from woman to woman, explains Dr. Neal Handel. "You definitely should rely on the opinion of your radiologist. There's no hard and fast rule that women should get both. The additional amount of information may not be worth doubling the radiation dose."

Some women may forego mammography because they are afraid it will increase the risk of rupture. This could delay a diagnosis of breast cancer, and worsen their prognosis if cancer is detected at a later stage. But, Dr. Michael Middleton, of the Department of Radiology at the University of California in San Diego, says, based on his experience and the fact that there is no research to the contrary, "We believe that it will be rare for a rupture of an intact implant to be *caused* by mammography under any circumstances, but that *exacerbation of existing* rupture by mammography is possible, especially if excessive force or improper technique is used."

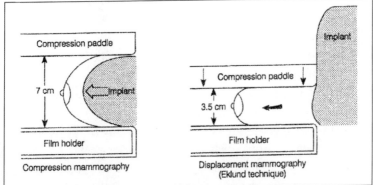

Compression mammography (left) sandwiches the breast and implant between the paddle and the film. Displacement mammography (right) shifts the implant back toward the chest, compressing the breast tissue only. The displacement technique may show more breast tissue than compression mammography in some women, but less in others.

In addition to detecting breast cancer, mammography can often identify an implant as being saline-filled or as being a double- or triple-lumen with an intact saline lumen. If you are unsure about whether your implants are silicone gel or saline, this would obviate the need for further imaging with, for example, MRI, assuming you did not have silicone-gel implants prior to your current implants. However, mammography is not useful for determining if an implant is ruptured, unless the silicone has escaped the scar capsule.

If you have severe contracture, you may want to have your implants removed because they could make it harder to detect breast cancer. As you age, your risk of breast cancer rises, and you may decide the benefits of having implants are no longer worth the risk. Another way to improve mammography may be to have your old implants removed, along with the hardened scar capsule, and replaced with newer implants (possibly behind the pectoral muscle) that are less likely to cause severe contracture. However, if an implant is placed behind the pectoralis muscle and it breaks or leaks, the silicone gel is harder to remove and more likely to destroy those muscles. And according to the manufacturers' own data and many surgeons' experiences, women who suffer from contracture once usually have it again if the implant is replaced. On the other hand, Handel measured the breast tissue visible by mammography before and after surgery to correct contracture; he found that "in most cases significantly more breast tissue" could be seen after the surgery. He feels that although no clinical studies prove that mammograms of saline-filled breasts are more accurately interpreted, saline implants are somewhat more radiolucent (permeable by the mammography X-ray beam), and it seems "prudent" to recommend them to women who are concerned.

Mammograms may be able to detect ruptures only if the gel has escaped outside the scar capsule (extracapsular), which occurred in about 26 percent of the implants evaluated in Middleton's 1998 study. MRI and ultrasound are better for detecting intracapsular ruptures, where the gel is still contained within the capsule. So, once your implants reach a certain age, or if you have symptoms that might indicate a rupture or leakage, it's time to add MRI, ultrasound, or both to your monitoring regime. Dr. Michael Middleton has performed over fifteen hundred MRIs on breast implants, and is a widely published researcher. He believes that MRI and ultrasound each have their own relative strengths and weaknesses. "In the proper setting, with adequate expertise, either can provide useful information to assist in the care of patients with breast implants, or those who have had them removed. Since both can be costly and time consuming, their utilization should be tailored to the needs of the individual patient," he says. He considers MRI and ultrasound to be "overlapping and complementary," with MRI being generally "better for implant evaluation, and ultrasound being better for soft-tissue silicone evaluation."

## Ultrasound (Sonography)

In certain women, ultrasound imaging may be advisable to detect ruptured silicone implants or to offer the possibility of detecting breast cancer early. Dr. Paul Striker reminds us that "in the best circumstances, mammography is 80 percent effective in detecting cancer—and that's in a woman whose breasts aren't dense. In a young woman with dense tissue it's less effective, and if she has an implant, it's even less effective." He recommends sonography as the only technique needed to monitor a gel implant in young women who are at lower risk for breast cancer; for women who are at increased risk for breast cancer, he recommends mammography, sonography, Doppler flow (a type of ultrasound), and transillumination (shining a light through the tissue). Most radiologists don't routinely do these tests, he says, but he believes this combination of four types of tests is needed to monitor implants and to detect breast cancer as early as possible. "Together these are 97 percent effective in detecting early cancer," Striker claims. Another technique involves using an endoscope—a slender, tubelike instrument inserted through a small incision in the breast, with which you can "explore the capsule and the intracapsular area" and "see disruptions and droplets of silicone outside the envelope."

Physicians at the Magee Women's Hospital Breast Care Center, in Pittsburgh, report that sonography detected even small implant leaks that failed to show up on a mammogram. Sonography also detected silicone in lymph nodes in the armpit, which mammography cannot do, and it was able to distinguish true leaks, which may require removal of the implant, from deformities in the implant, which may only require monitoring. Another group of researchers studied the sonograms of sixteen patients with nineteen ruptured silicone-gel implants (ruptures were confirmed at surgery in seventeen cases and by mammography and biopsy in the other two). Mammography revealed sixteen of the nineteen ruptures, and sonography showed seventeen of the nineteen ruptures. Sonography also detected masses of silicone that had entered the surrounding breast tissue and axilla (armpit tissue) in ten of the seventeen; in two of the ruptured implants, it detected the extruded portions only.

## Magnetic Resonance Imaging (MRI)

MRI causes silicone to appear brighter than the surrounding tissues. In 1998 Michael Middleton published the results of his study in which he used MRI to image 1,626 single-lumen silicone breast implants. In his hands, the sensitivity for rupture was 74 percent and specificity was 98 percent. To find an institution in your geographical area that is capable of delivering the quality of care necessary, Dr. Middleton advises you to talk to support groups, and then to contact the facilities and ask the following questions:

- Ask about the equipment; make sure it is state of the art. In Middleton's opinion, it should be a 1.5 tesla scanner, fast spin echo or its equivalent, and a dedicated breast coil operating in unilateral mode.

- Ask about the radiologists' experience. How many cases have they imaged? What is their sensitivity rate (ability to detect abnormalities), their specificity rate (ability to distinguish between silicone and tissue masses), and their ability to detect small leaks?

Middleton, who is considered one of the best interpreters of MRIs in the country, says he embraces a different point of view from many other radiologists. Others may claim a sensitivity rate of 95 percent or so, but Middleton feels that is because they do not realize they are missing what he calls microleaks or microruptures. When an implant with a microrupture is removed, he explains, it will have a thin layer of gel on the outside, which is attributed to gel bleed. Bleed consists only of oil, but a microrupture allows gel to escape in addition to oil, and he feels this may cause harm. "They miss this with their MRI, and they count it as a 'negative' [finding]," he says. "They don't pay attention to this during surgery, and if there is a small leak, they should call that an error." When Middleton finds a microrupture that his machine missed, he calls it a false negative. "My sensitivity is between 82 and 86 percent. This happens because the amount is simply too small for our MRI to detect; out of every one hundred implants we remove that we call negative, five will be positive or at a minimal level. I count those against me." He feels that other radiologists are not counting leakage; they are only counting gross rupture, either intracapsular or extracapsular. "It takes the right equipment, attitude, and experience. Many have the equipment; they just don't spend the time, or they don't think it's important."

## Other Tests

No single test or series of tests definitively diagnoses silicone-related disorders. However, there are a number of blood tests that some clinicians believe may be useful in detecting either excess silicone in the blood (indicating leakage or rupture) or other substances that could indicate silicone-related immune or autoimmune disorders. Several groups of researchers have reported antisilicone antibodies, but others have tried and failed to detect an immunologic response to silicone implants. These, along with a careful history, physical exam, and imaging techniques, may help you and your doctors make decisions about treatment. However, all of these blood tests are still experimental and controversial. None of them have been approved by the FDA, and many mainstream scientists dismiss them as worthless.

If you have polyurethane foam–coated implants, you can have your urine (and if breast-feeding, your breast milk) tested for TDA, the carcinogen released when the foam breaks down. Ask your physician to contact Aegis Laboratories at (615) 255-2400 (info@ aegislabs.com), or National Medical Service at (215) 657-4900.

The fact that we have no good way to monitor silicone-gel implants for bleed, leakage, and rupture frightens many of us—and angers many of us, too. The woman with undetected ruptured implants, whom we met in Chapter 4, says:

> I want to tell women that even though they're taking tests and their doctors are telling them there's nothing wrong, you still have to be concerned. There's no way that I can be the only one who's walking around with leaking implants and no indications. I had mammograms every year. Twice a year I had my breasts examined by my gynecologist. I even had a sonogram. I have been paying as much attention to this as I possibly could. Fortunately, I had complete medical coverage.
>
> No matter how wonderful women's doctors are and no matter how much confidence they have in them—they don't know. Nobody knows what's going on. It's a matter of faith at this point.

## Capsulotomy

Once capsular contraction has occurred, only one option exists: surgery, either to break up the capsule (*capsulotomy*) or to remove the capsule in its entirety (*capsulectomy*, discussed below).

In the past, capsular contraction of an implant placed in front of the muscle was treated by putting strong pressure on the implant (a procedure known as *closed capsulotomy*), which broke up the hardened tissue temporarily. This is no longer recommended, as it may increase the risk of implant rupture.

An *open capsulotomy*, although it is surgery, does not remove the scar tissue. In this procedure the surgeon may cut a larger pocket for the implant and replace it. If the implant was located above the muscle originally, replacing it below the muscle may help prevent another scar capsule from forming. Some surgeons also feel that using a textured saline implant may help, although there is some evidence that textured implants are harder to remove during explantation.

## Should You Remove or Replace Your Implants?

In the past, obvious rupture and unacceptable hardening were the major reasons for removing implants and, sometimes, the scar capsule; implants were usually put back in place or replaced with new implants. The FDA still states that you should not have intact implants removed if you are having no physical problems, because of the risks of the surgery. But the list of "problems," both known and suspected, has grown longer, and now we must also factor in our feelings of anxiety and doubt about the safety of implants, and most surgeons recommend removing implants that are known to be—or, because of their age, are likely to be—ruptured or leaking.

As a result of this anxiety, women today are having their implants surgically removed, or at least considering it, even if they are not suffering obvious implant-related problems. They are worried that the implants are time bombs that will cause problems in the future. How can you decide whether you should have your implants removed (*simple explantation*), and perhaps the scar capsule along with them (*capsulectomy*)? What factors enter into whether you should have them replaced, with either silicone-gel implants or saline implants?

### Reasons to Remove Implants and/or Scar Capsules

Most plastic surgeons and other experts agree implants should be removed (and replaced, if you wish) if:

◆ Your silicone implant has ruptured or leaked and is partially or wholly deflated (*intracapsular rupture*);

◆ Silicone gel has escaped from the implant envelope and the scar capsule and is detectable in your breast or elsewhere in your body (*extracapsular rupture*);

◆ Your saline implant has ruptured and has deflated, and you want it removed for aesthetic reasons and replaced with another. As an alternative, one plastic surgeon I spoke with has occasionally deflated the saline implant in the opposite breast of patients who have had augmentation. They preferred this solution, which involves puncturing the implant with a needle, in the doctor's office, to going through another surgery to remove the envelope and replace the implant to achieve symmetry;

◆ You have a spherical capsular contraction that is hard, painful, and deforms the breast. Some women do better if their gel implant is replaced with a saline or a textured implant, but others seem to form hard scar tissue no matter what. If you are one of these, you are probably better off having your implants removed, along with the scar tissue (capsulectomy), once and for all. If you have had breast reconstruction you may want to consider tissue transfer (see Chapter 3).

For women who are suffering from these easily diagnosed local problems, the benefits of explantation outweigh the risks, and the choice to remove the implants is fairly clear. But then there are gray areas, such as when a woman has systemic symptoms that could indicate a systemic disorder that might be attributed to implants. Here the decision is less obvious.

Because systemic symptoms that are associated with implants are so vague, ill defined, and impossible to diagnose definitively, there is no clear-cut way to determine if they are related to silicone and if removing an implant might help. However, removal of implants often seems to have a great impact on relieving symptoms. In fact, the improvement is so remarkable in 50 to 70 percent of women that this is the most powerful evidence that such a thing as silicone-related disease actually exists. Although some women feel better immediately after recuperating from the surgery, most take a long time to improve, and some actually feel worse before feeling better. It can take twelve months or more to begin to see improvement. Some women never feel completely well again; this may be because there is residual silicone in the body, or they have irreversible autoimmune disease, or their symptoms were unrelated to their implants. The questions are: Since not every woman improves after explantation, how are you to know if you will be one of them? And even if you did know you would improve, would you want to give up your implant?

As Dr. Frank Vasey points out, it is easy (and tempting) to attribute the symptoms to something else—overwork, stress, meno-

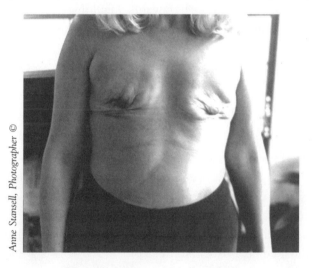

*Anne Stansell, Photographer ©*

*Explantation results vary greatly and depend on the reason for implantation, the severity of complications, the condition of the implant, the difficulty of removal, and the skills of the surgeon who removes them. This woman was told she was at high risk for breast cancer and was advised to have both her natural breasts removed to reduce her risk of the disease. She received silicone-gel implants but had an allergic reaction to them and they were removed and replaced with polyurethane-foam-coated implants. This second pair was also removed but not replaced. Not surprisingly, she says the results make her feel "mutilated." For good explantation results, see page 155.*

pause, and so on. Women who have had cancer and chemotherapy have long-term side effects to add to the daily stew of aches, pains, memory loss, and neurological symptoms. Vasey, who has treated hundreds of sick women with implants, notes in his book *The Silicone Breast Implant Controversy* (coauthored with Josh Feldstein) that "many women initially find it extremely difficult to accept that their chronic flulike symptoms, swollen glands, exhaustion, and other problems may be caused by silicone from their breast implants." In addition, so many women have been told by a series of doctors that "it's all in their head," they begin to believe it.

Vasey suggests that the cosmetic and psychological benefits of implants are so powerful that they keep women in denial, reluctant to even consider the possibility that in order to get healthy, they may have to give up their implants. I find this true even when we experience definite physical symptoms such as pain, tightness, and hardness. Most of us love(d) our implants. We got them because we wanted them; we were willing to undergo surgery for them—some of us many times. Symptoms, no matter how severe, have a tough time outweighing the desire to be whole again or to fulfill our society's standard of beauty. Dr. Harry Spiera, chief of rheumatology at Mount Sinai Medical Center, says, "There's a big difference between putting one in in the first place and having one removed. When women have put in an implant, they put it in for a reason; they've already gone through a procedure that carried a lot of emotional weight. Removing it isn't trivial. The only time I recommend removing it is if the person has an organ-threatening or life-threatening disease. And even then, removing the implant won't remove the silicone that has traveled."

Dr. Edward Knowlton, chief of plastic surgery at John Muir Hospital, says, "Before explantation, we want to make as sure as possible that this is the reason that she's sick, because it sets in gear a whole set of consequences once she gets her implants out. If she's had reconstruction, she may want to do tissue transfer— and this may be unnecessary. For the woman who's had augmentation, her breasts will be flat and droopy—it's a very emotional issue."

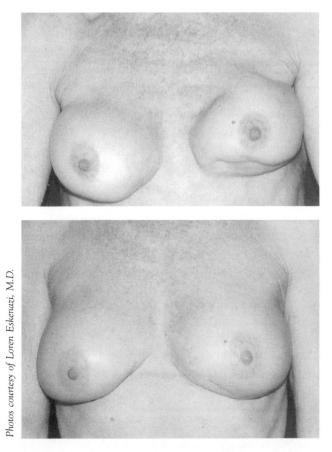

*Photos courtesy of Loren Eskenazi, M.D.*

**Top:** *Capsular contracture of silicone-gel implants.* **Bottom:** *After removal of implants and replacement with saline-filled implants.*

He further believes, "A doctor should consider talking to the patient about the option of removing the implant, especially if the patient got nondescript symptoms some time after implantation. I have a feeling there may be some people who fall through the cracks and who may benefit from exchanging the implants for saline or removing them altogether. It probably won't ameliorate their symptoms, but these people suffer so much, it's reasonable to try."

So far we have been talking about physical problems, as opposed to emotional pain. But what about the emotional anguish, the worry that the implants could cause health problems sooner or later? Should women with silicone-gel implants but no symptoms go through the pain, expense, and danger of having them removed? What about women with saline implants?

This woman found herself getting the runaround because her symptoms were written off as signs of menopause:

> I'd had implants a long time—I had mastectomies in 1972 because of fibrocystic breasts. I had local problems in the beginning, but then my general health began to deteriorate. I went from doctor to doctor, but because of my age, they all chalked it up to menopause. It was so exasperating—no one would listen to me. I had such extreme hot flashes, worse than anyone I knew; dry eyes and vagina that wouldn't respond to hormone therapy; migraine headaches; insomnia. I had one infection after another—a cold would always turn into a chest infection; I had bladder infections and was taking a lot of antibiotics. I had seven major infections in fifteen months! Allergies that I could never find the trigger for.
>
> The radiologist said my chest X ray showed emphysema and arterial pulmonary disease, but the pulmonary doctor said he didn't see anything. Yet I pursued it, and when I took a breathing test, I failed—my breathing tubes were constricted. Everything was getting worse, and I was getting more symptoms. I finally found a family practitioner who liked to diagnose. He wasn't sure my symptoms were implant related, but he was open-minded. He thought there could be a link in my case because there seemed to be no other explanation. He did the blood tests, and coordinated my care.

In my case, I did not have any systemic problems, but my implant was over sixteen years old. I had an MRI that indicated the saline portion of the double lumen had ruptured. The inner envelope containing the gel also was probably not in the greatest shape, and silicone had probably bled through the envelope and into the scar capsule. It could have been leaking already, or ready to rupture the next time I had sex or rolled onto my stomach. I agonized for years over whether I should remove it and replace it with a saline implant to prevent problems in the future. My plastic surgeon advised against it. This was—but may not still be—the prevailing point of view. Richard Jobe agreed:

> You can assume that after some years there will be some silicone in the breast capsule. But what the hell—it's been that way for the last five years, and it will be that way for the next twenty. Given that situation, I think there is no indication for removing the implant at the present time. I say someday you will probably have to have this implant out because it will leak. Or because we will have a splendid new implant that, for instance, will be more radiolucent. But right now, if silicone is confined to the breast capsule, I'm not convinced that it should be removed or replaced, because we have nothing on the market that's that much better to replace it with.

Dr. Striker advised me to leave well enough alone, too: "If you're not having any problems, the risk of surgery is probably greater than the risk of leaving it in."

Although there are still plastic surgeons who dismiss women's concerns—and even refuse to do explantation—an increasing number are taking a more compassionate, humanistic attitude. One plastic surgeon, a died-in-the-wool skeptic, said to me, "If it worries them on a daily basis, take the implants out. Period." Dr. Striker says he has had patients who have no problems with their implants whatsoever: "No contracture, no rupture, no symptoms—but they're worried. They say, 'I have a family history of cancer, I can't sleep at night—I've got to get it out, I feel the silicone is going to hurt me.' Psychologically those people are candidates for explantation, with or without exchange."

Dr. Spiera says, "Most people I've seen are fairly happy with their implants…but all the publicity is making people nervous as hell. I had a woman come see me; she said she loved her implants, she was happy and comfortable. But she asked me, 'Am I going to die? Am I going to get this?' And she was fine. I just don't know how to deal with it. I'm one of the people that started this and I feel very bad for these ladies. We just need much more data."

Knowlton recognizes the importance of perceived risk:

> If a woman feels, rightly or wrongly, that she has a time
> bomb in her chest and is losing sleep over it, she has the
> option to have the implant removed and perhaps replaced.
> There might be some gel in the capsule, and so a woman
> might feel the scar capsule also needs to be removed along
> with the implant. But she should bear in mind that this is a
> more extensive operation and may not be worth the extra
> risk; maybe just removing the implant would be the better
> choice.

If you are not overly worried, and if you do not have systemic symptoms, or if your local symptoms are bearable, there is no rush to remove your implants. You may never become ill. However, we now know that you can have leakage and rupture without symptoms, and that the older the implant is, the more likely it is that this has occurred, making surgery more difficult to perform.

It is advisable that you monitor your health and be aware of any subtle or slowly worsening sensations. Keep a journal of how you feel—note any aches and pains that occur in the absence of increased physical activity, fatigue that cannot be explained by anything specific, sleep problems, and so on. Symptoms of immune disease are so subtle and insidious you may not notice them until you look at a slowly building, overall pattern. Such symptoms require medical evaluation, whether you have implants or not.

Implants can cause symptoms that mimic other diseases, but sometimes symptoms can be brushed off as implant related when they are a sign of serious disease. Said one woman:

> Shortly after my implant surgery, I began having sharp pings
> on the side [of my chest] opposite my implant. My surgeon
> attributed it to stress on muscle or connective tissue due to
> the surgery. It would come and go, seemingly related to my
> exercise pattern. Two years ago, it flared up quite strongly,
> and I thought for sure it was a cancer recurrence. My life
> flashed before me, but the bone scan was normal. My
> internist diagnosed an inflammation of the cartilage between
> my ribs (cause unknown), and after applying ice (actually

bags of frozen peas) to the area, it eventually calmed down. It's probably due to all the anatomical yanking that my implant is imposing on my aging body. I continue to have those strange pings after some strenuous aerobic dance classes, and even after yoga. But at least I'm pretty sure it's not cancer.

A friend of this woman had a different tale to tell:

I've had all sorts of problems with my implants after reconstruction. Debilitating headaches, shoulder and neck aches, fatigue. When I started having pain in my sternum and collarbones, I attributed it to the implants as well. But my doctor eventually became concerned, and we had another bone scan ahead of schedule. Bad news: The cancer had recurred and was causing the pain, not the implants. I'd just had a normal scan less than a year before.

## Capsulectomy

People who believe in silicone-related disease recommend that the scar capsule be removed along with the implant. This is called removal *en bloc* (as a whole). Silicone gel bleeds into the tissue, and particles of the envelope may break off and become imbedded in the scar as well. Removing as much as possible will lessen the chance of silicone-related complications. However, removal of the scar capsule may require a larger incision than simple explantation, and may cause more pain, more bleeding, and more disfigurement.

Nancy Carteron, a rheumatologist in the San Francisco area, feels it is "absolutely imperative" to remove the scar capsule and send tissue to a lab that is experienced in silicone. She says the majority of physicians still do not believe there is a real association between silicone and illness; she has heard colleagues who are involved with evaluations of women make off-the-record remarks that they think women are just in the litigation for the money. "I had a patient who was very ill and didn't have her capsule out along with the implant. She's still symptomatic and I don't feel we did everything we can do for her, because we haven't taken the capsules out."

Loren Eskenazi, a San Francisco–area plastic surgeon, has become less skeptical of the association because "there are some people who have no other explanations for their problems other than silicone gel." Still, she says:

> Although it is more drastic surgery and usually requires general anesthesia, I always take out the capsule along with the implant. From a health point of view, I don't think it matters. But it matters to the lawyers and it matters to the patients. So I do it, unless it would harm the patient. For example, one woman had a bad infection. I removed just the implant, and went back to remove the capsule six months later when the infection had cleared up.

Several studies provide evidence that it's imperative to remove the scar capsule along with the implants. As mentioned in the previous chapter, the capsule is a catch-all for liquid, gel, and elastomer silicone particles and droplets, and tissue surrounding a silicone-gel implant contains on average 108,000 times more silicone than unexposed tissue. Even saline implants shed silicone from the envelope, and your capsule could contain eighty-three times more silicone than is normal. If not removed, the silicone left behind could continue to cause problems (or eventually begin to cause problems); if you replace your implants, presumably the silicone would continue to build up. Your body may reabsorb the capsule once the implant is removed. Or it may not, according to several studies. A 1998 study by W. Bradford Rockwell and colleagues found that in eight women the capsule persisted for up to seventeen years. In another study, published in 1995, N.S. Hardt and colleagues write that after explantation without capsulectomy "an uneventful resolution is not always the case, and several potential problems may arise from retained capsules." Possible consequences include a mass suspicious for cancer, dense calcifications that make it difficult to read mammograms, cystic masses, hematoma, and cysts filled with silicone. Dr. Douglas Shanklin, a pathologist, wrote:

There is a remarkably large body of medical and scientific literature…which emphatically shows the capsule is the site of illness. It is one thing to debulk the patient of silicone load by explantation, but unless the capsules come out at the same time, the immunopathic process will continue unabated. The standard is not whether something is usual or customary, but whether it is the correct and logical thing to do.

And Dr. Pierre Blais, a scientist who had been studying the interaction between medical materials and living tissue, writes, "It is well documented from case histories that removal and/or replacement of implants without exhaustive debridement of the prosthetic site leads to failure and post surgical complications." The list of undesirable consequences as a result of leaving in the capsule includes reformation of capsular contracture if the implants are replaced. And when implants are not replaced, the capsule may collapse and visually disappear, but eventually fill with extracellular debris; it may shrink and calcium salts collect, making mammography difficult. As time goes by, nodules may form, mimicking cancer and leading to surgical biopsies. Needle biopsies are not advisable, according to Blaise, because this could release hazardous material and infectious agents encased in the capsule. Left untouched, the capsule is permeable and may periodically release microorganisms into the surrounding breast tissue. The capsule may continue to evolve and become thicker, forming granulomas or causing abscesses or solid "tumor-like structures" to form. If you would like to read more about explantation and the compelling reasons to remove your implant(s) en bloc, visit http://explantation.com.

## Obtaining a Pathology Report

After explantation and capsulectomy, you may want to send the implant and tissue to a special lab for analysis. If you are concerned that your implant has deteriorated or want to know how or why it ruptured, or if you want your scar tissue studied to see whether it has reacted with the silicone, ask to take it with you after removal. Make your wishes known in writing. You have every right to do this, since the implant is your property. Before turning it over to you, your doctor may want independent documentation of its condition, in case there is a lawsuit later on. Implants and tissue must be packaged and transported following strict procedures. You need to request before explantation that this be done; discuss this with your surgeon or contact the support groups listed in the Resources section and ask if anyone there can recommend a lab.

Saul Puszkin, a pathologist at New York's Mount Sinai School of Medicine, has analyzed the gel inside the implant, the capsule, and any other tissue removed with the implant from fifteen hundred patients. He looks for inflammation, pathological changes, and infiltration of foreign materials such as silicone and polyurethane. He says he wants to see "how the patient reacted to the implant. I analyze the blood serum to see if there are antibodies and what they have been formed to—is it the nervous system? Does she have headaches that could be explained by the antibodies?"

Carteron says, "Most pathology labs don't know how to handle it. They don't want to spend the extra money, and the insurance company is not going to pay, or the person isn't going to want to pay for the detailed evaluation that one would need to definitively decide whether there was a silicone reaction or not." That's why it's necessary to use a specialty lab.

## Risks of Implant Removal and Capsulectomy

Since implant removal requires surgery, patients run the usual risks of infection, bleeding, and reaction to the anesthesia. They also will experience postoperative pain and will need time to recuperate.

Ironically, surgery also poses the risk of causing the implant to burst, creating more problems than if it had been left alone. In addition, women take the chance that they are removing something that might have lasted for many more years.

Although after explantation women may feel relieved about being implant-free, they may also experience mixed emotions. The Doctor's Company, a malpractice insurer, has supplied its plastic-surgeon subscribers with a special consent form for breast-implant removal. It advises patients that removal may result in a strong negative impact on their physical appearance (including significant loss of breast volume, distortion, and appearance worse than before the initial augmentation); severe psychological effects, including depression; loss of interest in sexual relations for themselves or their partners; and scarring that may prevent future reconstruction. This consent form of necessity overstates the case; however, plastic surgeons find that although some patients are emotionally relieved after having implants removed, others are upset over the results and sometimes decide to have them put back in.

Removing an intact implant is generally not much more difficult than inserting it; it may in fact be easier because the surgeon does not need to create the pocket. The procedure can become more involved when the implant has a polyurethane-foam coating, has a hard capsule surrounding it, has ruptured, or is eroded and fragile. In these cases, the surgeon may need to remove embedded tissue and muscle.

## Making the Explantation Decision

Before you take such a drastic step as explantation, get all the information you can. Consult with the appropriate medical specialists—this may include rheumatologists, neurologists, and plastic surgeons—to discuss options and evaluate your implants. Michael Middleton, a radiologist, says, "It's especially important to have a family practitioner or internist to guide the patient through this maze of specialists. If you can find someone like that, he's worth his weight in gold."

Middleton also recommends consulting with a psychologist. "These are normal women who are going through heavy stress, and just like a cancer patient or someone who has experienced the death of someone close to them, they would benefit in many cases from therapy or someone to talk to." He points out that "a woman may be reluctant to admit that she needs therapy, when she has been seeing doctors who have been telling her that her symptoms are all in her head. It also may look bad legally." In such a case, support groups are another option for hashing out one's thoughts and feelings. Plastic surgeons usually have one or two psychologists they refer patients to in cases where doubt exists as to whether the procedure is advisable from a psychological point of view. Sharyn Higdon Jones, a psychotherapist, has written a short guide for women titled "Five Important Issues to Explore When Considering Implantation—or Explantation," which is included in Appendix A.

Middleton, who has expertise in imaging breast implants, believes MRI and other imaging techniques play a role in helping a woman make a decision about explantation, although they are only "one piece of the puzzle."

Others, such as Eskenazi, believe it is a waste of money to undergo an MRI to see if an implant has ruptured, because "only if you're having symptoms do you need to take out your implant, regardless of whether it's ruptured or not. If you believe that gel causes disease, then you must believe that an intact implant causes disease as well as a ruptured one. I believe it can happen—but I also believe it's rare."

While Middleton says it is true that rupture and leaks do not necessarily correlate with symptoms—only 25 percent of his cases turn out to have ruptured implants and, he says, "we have a pretty sick group"—he also believes this is a valuable piece of information.

> Some women will ask, 'Why should I get an MRI, when I can have the operation and a diagnosis at the same time?' The problem is the operation is many thousands of dollars, and [MRI] is a noninvasive method of evaluation that may prevent an operation and the accompanying complications.

Middleton describes the case of a woman around thirty years old who was in an automobile accident. She and her plastic surgeon were sure her implants had ruptured through seat-belt injury. He scheduled her for emergency surgery, but Middleton gave her an MRI the night before. The MRI revealed she had sustained neither leak nor rupture. She canceled her emergency surgery. Middleton notes that she eventually rescheduled an elective explantation with saline replacements. "The advantage," he says, "was there were no surprises after the surgery, with the implants coming out intact." The surgeon modified the surgery to be appropriate for intact implants: He made a smaller incision, with less anesthesia; she avoided hospitalization and saved money. "Because the decision was based on all available data," says Middleton, "she was a satisfied customer."

Once you have all the medical information available, you can decide whether leaving your implants in is a risk you are willing to take. Recognize that you are making your decision in light of the best information available at the time, so when you look back years later, you won't regret your decision. As Middleton says, "We always make decisions in all aspects of life on inadequate data; you just need to take your best shot."

Make sure you thoroughly understand the procedure before agreeing to it, and the specific risks in your case. As with any surgical procedure, it is usually recommended that you get a second opinion before proceeding. Any board-certified plastic surgeon should be able to perform an explantation, and you should have no trouble finding one.

Be aware, however, that some doctors may be reluctant to do the surgery. Carteron, the rheumatologist, admits that for someone without symptoms, she would be "hard-pressed as a medical practitioner to recommend that you have your implants removed now, given the ongoing controversy, the risk of the surgery and anesthesia, and the psychological issues."

In her experience, women who received implants for augmentation are less likely to have them removed than women who had implants for reconstruction. Women with local symptoms "tend to be able to tolerate a lot of local discomfort before they have them removed or replaced." As far as women with systemic symptoms are concerned, Carteron has examined women who have been sick for a number of years, are out of work, have marriages that have fallen apart, have no other explanation for their symptoms, or feel that what they have experienced is consistent with what others have experienced. She says, "About 80 percent of these women with systemic symptoms have their implants taken out—or would, if they could afford it."

For many women, deciding whether or not to remove their implants is an unsolvable dilemma; for others, the decision is clear because they have no other options, no other possible explanation for their symptoms. Here is what four women have to say about their decision-making processes:

❖ I'm not sure that there's a connection between my symptoms and my implants. I'm not deathly ill, but I'm convinced that these things have a shelf life and I'm at the upper end of mine. I'd like to have a child, but I'm concerned about the ill effects [of the implants] on my baby. My doctor advises me to have my implants removed before I become pregnant. But what if I do that and I can't become pregnant? Or if I lose the baby—I'm in my early forties, and I've already had one miscarriage. For now, I just don't sleep on my stomach because I'm afraid they'll rupture or that stuff will ooze out when I put pressure on them.

❖ Right now I'd characterize my feelings as either denial or judicious caution. My mood swings, depending on my latest experience, on what I hear—these things stir me from the denial mode. But most of the time I feel that I'll be okay. The symptoms I'm suffering are mild, but I resent them bitterly. Because one of the tools of my recovery from cancer may be a source of disease. Because it's only now being revealed that these things weren't tested. There's a lot of psychological pain in finding out that you might have to lose your breast all over again.

❖ These things creep up on you, but I started noticing symptoms while I was on vacation in Europe. I had trouble walking because my knees were so sore. Now I have trouble starting to walk when I get out of the car. But then again, my mom has pretty bad arthritis too. I also feel fatigued—but all the stress of worrying about my implants could just be wearing me out. I just had a sonogram of my implants—it was "suspicious" for rupture—and they're only four years old! I want to have them out soon, and not wait to get to the point where I'm really sick.

◆  I was getting worse and worse—sicker, with more infections every year. I had so many things going wrong with me. I could check off about a third of the symptoms on the list of silicone-related symptoms: allergies, infections, swollen achy joints, my chest X ray showed the beginnings of emphysema. Although my implants weren't that hard, something was definitely wrong with my immune system. I finally had an MRI, which showed that both my implants were ruptured. Although most of my blood tests came back normal, the thyroid was off the chart. That did it—with no other possible explanation for my symptoms, I decided I would try taking the implants out. Then began the search for a surgeon who would remove them. Three months later, they came out. I noticed a difference within a couple of weeks—less achy, my insomnia is better, my head doesn't pulse with headaches, the last cold I got didn't turn into pneumonia, and my digestive problems have improved. My arthritic thumb joint will probably not get better—my rheumatologist said it might get worse. I'm hoping that the emphysema stabilizes. I still need to keep antibiotics on hand, and I take an antidepressant and thyroid medication. But I'm hopeful I'll continue to improve.

## Who Pays?

Be sure to discuss beforehand the fee for explantation. Some physicians demand the entire fee in advance; others may waive the entire fee (which, incidentally, could "help diminish the risk of a dissatisfied patient" according to the Doctor's Company). The fee for removing the implant alone may differ from that for also removing the capsule surrounding the implant.

Some insurance companies cover removal of implants; many do not.

## Making the Decision about Replacement, Tissue Transfer, Uplift, or Further Diagnosis

If you have two silicone-gel implants (because of either augmentation or reconstruction after a double mastectomy), only one may need removal because of rupture or severe contracture. Discuss the pros and cons of replacing just one with a saline implant. You may decide to replace both, or remove both, because a saline implant is unlikely to match the silicone implant in look or feel.

This woman's ruptured silicone-gel implants were removed, and she opted to have them replaced with saline-filled implants:

> When I had these done I wasn't even told I had the option of putting saline in. My surgeon said they were safe and good for the rest of your life. That's what they knew in those days. I'm angry that I had to go through this a second time and then to find out what was going on in my body.... You might ask why I had saline implants put back in. It was spooky to put them in, because the casing is still silicone, and there are no guarantees about that, either. But I'm a woman. I liked the way my body looked with implants. I never regretted having them. With all the anger I feel, I wouldn't want to be without them now. We all like to believe what we want to believe. We all want happy endings. We don't think we'll be the one who has breast cancer, or the one whose implant leaks.

In spite of the potential drawbacks, many women are glad to be rid of their worrisome implants and choose not to replace them with anything. Others choose to have new silicone implants or saline implants. Discuss this and other options with your surgeon. Your decision depends, in part, on the reason you are having implants removed. There may be specific medical reasons you should not have another implant, such as the likelihood of capsular contracture. Replacing a silicone-gel implant with a saline-filled implant may give you more peace of mind if you are thus far symptom-free. However, since saline implants have silicone envelopes, they may still pose problems for women who are hyper-sensitive to silicone.

Dr. Harry Spiera says, "If you think silicone could be causing problems, it doesn't make sense to replace them with saline, because you're still putting the silicone shell in the body. We don't know whether it's the shell or the gel that might be causing problems."

It is true that saline implants are not trouble- or worry-free. But they do offer certain advantages over silicone gel (for example, they are less likely to cause contracture), and if it is the gel that is causing problems, at least you have eliminated one possibility. For some women it is a clear choice, but in other cases, Eskenazi says she has to determine whether a person can "tolerate" switching to saline:

> For women who say, 'Gee, I think I want them out. Could they be causing my tiredness?' but are attached to their body shape, I'll convert them to saline. If their symptoms are severe, they have documented disease, it's disabling their lives, I tell patients to take them out and not put anything in. There's always the very, very small chance that they will have a problem with saline as well—either physical or psychological.

Other women are less sanguine about saline:

◆ I'm dragging my feet because my symptoms aren't serious and I'm hoping I can hold out until something better than saline comes out. I'm concerned about saline—I don't think it's the answer because of the dangers of infection and deflation—why should I exchange silicone which may or may not cause problems for something that might need replacing again and again?

◆ I waited after I had my implants out to decide about whether I'd have the TRAM flap. I wanted to see if I'd get better, and I did. I never considered saline—after having silicone implants for twenty-four years, I just didn't want anything else foreign in there. My body is not a Zip-Loc bag that you can keep opening up and putting things into and out of.

❖    I wouldn't have my silicone implants replaced with saline—they didn't know the problems with silicone, and five years from now what if they find there are problems with saline too? I don't want to exchange one cloud of doubt for another. I'm fifty-two years old—I don't want to be locked into replacing them again when I'm sixty or seventy. I think I'm better off doing a TRAM flap now while I'm healthy. I want it to be over and done with so I can get on with my life—rather than thinking about them all the time. But if I can't use my own tissue, I would just talk myself into getting used to living with nothing—which is what my family would prefer anyway.

Surgeons have seen a huge increase in the number of women who are interested in tissue-transfer surgery for reconstruction—particularly the TRAM flap, involving tissue from the abdomen—even though it is a very complicated, expensive operation.

For women who had their implants for augmentation, Eskenazi says:

They need to know that in addition to explantation they can have an uplift to correct drooping breasts, and they will often have a better appearance than they did with their implants if their implants were hard. Their breasts are smaller, perkier, softer. They look more natural and in proportion to their body. So women should ask their surgeons if they are a candidate for this procedure, either at the time of explantation or after.

Dr. Eskenazi does this procedure at the same time as the explantation, but she says many surgeons are reluctant to do it concurrently because of the issue of maintaining an adequate blood supply to the nipple. If the surgeon does not want to do it, Eskenazi recommends going to another surgeon for a second opinion.

In Dr. Middleton's experience, about half the women who have MRIs to look for rupture or leakage have their implants removed (regardless of the results). Of the women whose MRIs indicate rupture or leakage (20 to 25 percent), around 95 percent have their implants removed. Of those who take them out, 30 percent replace

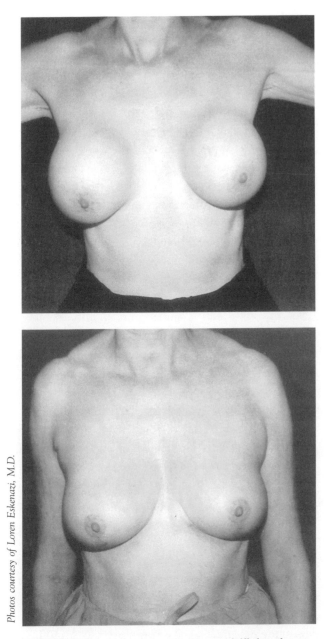

**Top:** *Capsular contracture with silicone-gel-filled implants.*
**Bottom:** *After removal of implants and a breast lift (mastopexy).*

*Photos courtesy of Loren Eskenazi, M.D.*

silicone with saline, 30 percent have a mastopexy on the explanted breasts, and 30 percent simply take the implants out and do nothing further. The last 10 percent are equally divided among those who replace the implant with another silicone implant, have a conventional flap, and have a free flap. Middleton says that of the women who leave them in, half are "kind of sick" but unwilling to take the big step of explantation, and the other half are reassured by the MRI and glad they "get to keep their implants."

If you decide to remove your silicone-gel implants because they have ruptured and the gel was found outside the capsule, you may want to have an MRI or a mammogram after the surgery to see if any residual pockets of silicone are left in the chest area. This is especially important if you still have symptoms. According to Project Impact, an education and advocacy group, some women have found their health improved after having the residual silicone removed.

Dr. Susan Kolb, a plastic surgeon and holistic health practitioner, believes that if a woman has silicone-gel implants and they are five years old or older, they need to be removed. However, five years may be a little extreme, and others feel that seven to ten years might be a more reasonable point to consider removal. If a woman has been in a car accident or other traumatic event, Kolb says, she needs to realize that this may cause a rupture, and she needs to be more vigilant. She advises women to have implants taken out by a plastic surgeon—not a general surgeon—who does explants regularly. "And," she adds, "it should be someone who believes that silicone can cause illness, because otherwise they may not be as careful in removing it."

She notes that many women get worse after explantation, as she did. Although she believes she had good surgeons, and she told them what she wanted them to do, "they did not listen. The surgeons did not take out all of the capsules, and they didn't take care not to spill silicone in me." Because she was sick and failed to improve after explantation, she was moved to devise a systemic program to help herself as well as the many patients who come to her for explantation (see below).

## Systemic Treatments

Many women have tried different types of treatment protocols for the various symptoms they believe are related to their implants. As one "implant survivor" says, "What works for one may not work for the next," and she suggests visiting a website where women share treatments that have worked for them. One such site is: http://community-1.webtv.net/lany25/LifeAfterBreast0/.

According to Nancy Carteron, no bona fide treatment is available for silicone-induced disease besides implant removal and capsulectomy. She says some people have found benefit from antidepression medication, primarily those in the serotonin uptake inhibitor group, such as Zoloft and Prozac. Their depression may be due to chronic pain and having gone through a number of surgeries, or it may be part of the same syndrome as sleep disturbance and neurological symptoms such as memory loss and other cognitive abnormalities. In Carteron's experience, "People who have a lot of pain also feel better on this medicine. For the pain and fatigue of fibromyalgia, we use a low dose of Elavil [an antidepressant]."

She also recommends that people "take care of themselves, to allow their own immune system to be as strong as possible: diet, exercise, stress reduction—all those things that are easy to say and hard to do." She does not recommend specific herbs or alternative medicines.

We do not yet know whether silicone is eventually excreted and, if so, whether this process can be accelerated. According to Dr. Frank Vasey, animal studies indicate that silicone is excreted in the urine; in addition, some women with implants suffer from a painful bladder condition called interstitial cystitis that may indicate silicone is excreted in humans. "This is actually encouraging," observes Carteron, "[T]he hope would be that with time, the body load would be less and less. Perhaps one can then look at developing binding agents that would then increase excretion." The best bet for now is to keep yourself as healthy as possible, thereby optimizing your normal excretory process.

Dr. Susan Kolb, the plastic surgeon who is also board certified in holistic medicine, says that explantation is the cornerstone of her program, because it is necessary to get rid of the source of the problem. But she follows this up with a holistic protocol designed to detoxify the body of silicone and heavy metals. The program also modulates the immune system—some aspects need to be calmed and others may need to be stimulated. Components of the program include:

- A diet that avoids animal protein and emphasizes fresh fruits, vegetables, and whole grains, as well as plenty of filtered or distilled water

- An exercise program of walking and stretching

- Supplements, including antioxidants and anti-inflammatory nutrients

- Herbs

- Stress management

- Medication for systemic bacterial or fungal infection

- Intravenous nutritional therapy and therapy for candidiasis; chelation therapy for heavy metals

- Detoxification techniques such as fasting, colon cleansing, and nutritional supplements

- Glandular therapy

- Enzyme therapy

She emphasizes that the program is individualized; it varies from person to person. It is not meant to be done all at one time, and it also changes over time for each person. She admits that her program "isn't the be-all and end-all. More research needs to be done. I just talked to experts all over the country and I have some ideas."

She has seen over a thousand women who were ill, and she says that most do improve on her program, but she does not know how long they will need to be on the program or whether they will continue to improve. She has been on the program herself since 1997, when she had her silicone implants removed. She says that the longer a silicone implant has been ruptured or leaking, the longer it takes for a woman to get better. She warns that in most cases, you can't do a program like this on your own. You need to have professional care, a complete physical exam, and lab tests; and your doctor needs to have a knowledge of implants, and be able to diagnose heavy-metal poisoning. She says your best bet is a holistic doctor; while not every holistic practitioner is familiar with silicone, many are. (See "Treatment Clinics," in Resources, for a list of holistic doctors, with their contact information.)

## Caveat Emptor (Let the Buyer Beware)

Just as we must be savvy about implants to begin with, we must be careful when seeking medical treatment for disorders that might be due to our implants. In the early 1990s, CNN's weekly news magazine *Fire and Fury* aired a story that asked, "Are there medical hucksters cashing in on women's panic about implants for their personal profit?" The show concluded yes, women are preyed upon by the very doctors they are turning to for help. They found "a thriving cottage industry of doctors, labs, and treatment centers that were selling dubious science and questionable diagnoses and treatments." They interviewed patients and doctors who said they knew of women who were being misled by opportunists—labs that charge between one thousand and twenty-five hundred dollars for experimental tests of unproven value. (Two pathologists I called while researching this book strongly urged me to have my implant taken out immediately and sent to them for analysis; one offered to waive his usual eighteen-hundred-dollar fee.)

CNN focused in particular on one doctor from a well-respected medical college. He admitted earning three hundred thousand dollars a year treating breast-implant patients; he says he has good results, but did not supply proof. Although some patients called him a hero, one patient and several of his colleagues called him a huckster. His colleagues were unconvinced that he was treating silicone-induced illness—or that his patients even had this condition. One patient of his had spent ninety thousand dollars so far on her treatment: gamma globulin, prednisone (a steroid), Cytoxan (a cancer chemotherapy drug), and an experimental drug that is injected into her stomach. She had not yet improved, but she said the doctor told her that if she did not have the treatment, she would get worse quickly and perhaps die. Another patient, who had spent sixty thousand dollars, said the treatments were "frightening" but that women were desperate and "looking so much for someone to say 'I can help you' that we want to believe he can help us."

The lesson is this: Exercise caution when consulting with practitioners who promise or suggest they can treat implant-related disease. The treatments are usually experimental, with little formal data to back them up. Even credentialed physicians can legally offer treatment that is unproven and experimental—and often extremely costly—as long as it has been FDA approved for some purpose.

# 7

# Alternatives to Implants

Before making any decisions regarding implants, it is wise to explore the alternatives. You need to know what's available and their pluses and minuses, just as you need to know the potential benefits and risks of breast implants. It is also a good idea to familiarize yourself with your options before you decide to remove implants you already have.

## Replacing a Breast after Mastectomy

Wanting a reconstruction after mastectomy is a healthy emotional response for many women, but it is not a procedure for everyone. Especially with the current uncertainty about the safety of implants, you may be less inclined to undergo anymore surgery, pain, or expense. Or you may want to choose an alternative that will temporarily fill your needs; doing so could give you more time to think about whether you want reconstruction and to see what new information becomes available.

Three basic alternatives to implants are available for women who have had mastectomies: no breast replacement, a breast prosthesis worn outside the body, and surgeries that involve using the woman's own tissue to reconstruct a breast.

How you feel about the various alternatives will depend on many factors, including the size and shape of your remaining breast, whether you have had a single or double mastectomy, your feelings about your body, your lifestyle, your sexual relationships and preferences, the stage of your disease, and your prognosis. Cost will also be a factor, especially if you have inadequate or no medical insurance.

## No Replacement

Some women feel comfortable with their bodies after mastectomy and do nothing about replacing their breasts. They choose clothing carefully to disguise the surgery, or make no attempt to hide it at all, reasoning that if it bothers other people, it's the other person's problem. Women who choose this route sometimes do so as a way of expressing their feminist or spiritual beliefs; some don't want to go through further surgery; others feel that this acceptance of their appearance is a natural and healthy response after the trauma of dealing with the cancer.

In her book *Tree*, Deena Metzger traces the journey that led her to find a way to live with the loss of her breast that involved neither reconstruction nor prosthesis. She admits that at first the idea of asymmetry bothered her. Later, she came to feel that "Perhaps it is not so bad to look like an Amazon. We are new kinds of warriors." Nevertheless, she attempted reconstruction at one point, in the hope that she "was not going to have to worry about whether she was funny-looking anymore," but the surgery was unsuccessful due to "mechanical difficulties." By the end of the book, she arrives at a healing and liberating idea for dealing with the scar on one side of her chest: a tattoo of a branch of a tree, which for her symbolizes the life force. Another breast cancer patient, who was in her early thirties when she was diagnosed, never really considered reconstruction. "Why would I want to go through more surgery?" she asks. She wears a prosthesis under her clothing, except when she swims or body surfs. Then she goes without, and sometimes she even goes topless, proud of her statuesque body and of her beauty, which is not diminished by her lack of symmetry.

Susan Love, a breast surgeon, writes in *Dr. Susan Love's Breast Book*, "It's wonderful to have the self-confidence to feel comfortable without the appearance of a breast, but most of us are products of our culture and need to feel that we are cosmetically acceptable to the outside world." She also points out that there may be a price to pay for not looking "normal," and that if you opt for this solution, you may want to wear a prosthesis, at least on the job.

"Going without" 24/7 may pose medical problems. Our bodies are designed to wear equal weight on the chest, and women who forgo a breast form, in particular, may eventually suffer neck, shoulder, and back problems. Large-breasted women may especially suffer from the imbalance, but they are not alone. Although I was by no means well endowed, the shoulder and back pain I experienced after my mastectomy vanished a day or two after I began wearing a high-quality prosthesis.

## External Breast Prostheses

An external prosthesis is the most popular alternative to a breast implant because, in clothing, it does a pretty good job of restoring the appearance of a breast. Finding the right prosthesis can go a long way toward helping women feel physically and psychologically comfortable.

Most women receive a temporary prosthesis in the hospital, often through an American Cancer Society's Reach to Recovery program volunteer. These prostheses are usually made of a soft fluffy material that the woman can adjust to approximate her own size and shape. They are comfortable, and look fine in loose-fitting clothing. Some women continue to use fluffy material, but most are dissatisfied with the feel or appearance and go on to buy a regular breast form.

When considering a prosthesis, wait until you are physically and emotionally ready to shop around for the one that is best for you. Breast prostheses and mastectomy bras are sold in surgical-supply stores, in the underwear departments of large department stores, by mail order, and in lingerie and corset shops, which often also carry specially designed sportswear and attractive lingerie for women with mastectomies.

To find a supplier, look under "brassieres," "prostheses," or "surgical appliances" in the yellow pages, or call or visit your local chapter of the American Cancer Society or a breast-care center. Or shop online; just go to your favorite search engine—such as yahoo.com or google.com—and type in "breast prosthesis."

The American Cancer Society's Reach to Recovery program in New York City provided me with a list of local prosthesis sources. They also showed me a filing-cabinet drawer full of sample prostheses to demystify the product and to give me a preview of what my options would be when I was ready to shop. True to my personality, the thought and the sight of a filing cabinet full of breasts struck me as hilariously funny and put me in the perfect mood to proceed to the mastectomy boutique. Some ACS units set a specific time and day for regularly scheduled presentations of options after mastectomy. Others will set up appointments for one-on-one consultation and counseling.

Many shops that sell prostheses are staffed or owned by women who have had mastectomies themselves, so you are likely to be dealing with someone who is sensitive and understanding. You might want additional emotional support, though, so consider bringing a close friend or family member. Prostheses are made of a variety of materials. Many are made of a rubbery form of silicone, and most women find that silicone best approximates the weight and feel of a natural breast. Some types of prostheses are filled with tiny beads that let the breast move in a way that more closely resembles that of a natural breast. The outside may be soft fabric, polyurethane, or clear silicone "skin."

Prostheses come in a variety of sizes and vary in weight and firmness. They are available to fit either the right or left side. Most women looking for a prosthesis have had a modified radical mastectomy, and many models are made to fit this surgery. But you can also find prostheses that cover a lot—to fill gaps in tissue left by radical mastectomies—or a little—such as those designed to fill out breasts that have had extensive lumpectomies. Prostheses that impart the most natural look to partial mastectomies or lumpectomies are usually a type of silicone shell with a built-in nipple. These may also be preferred when implant surgery results in a lopsided chest, with one breast smaller than the other. Some models have a nipple included, or you may buy a separate nipple. These are also used by women who have breast-only reconstruction without a surgically reconstructed nipple.

Insurance companies cover at least part of the cost of prostheses; a prescription from your physician helps facilitate the process. If the cost is a problem (a high-quality off-the-shelf breast form costs between $175 and $300), the American Cancer Society and some breast cancer–support organizations may be able to provide you with one from their supply of donated products.

## No-Bra Adhesives

Most women rely on a bra of some sort to keep their prosthesis in place. Others swear by adhesives that allow them to wear a prosthesis without resorting to special bras or swimwear. In fact, an adhesive can give you the freedom to go braless or to wear strapless or other style-conscious or revealing clothing.

Until recently, only liquid surgical adhesive was available, which needed to be removed and reapplied daily. New designs employ an adhesive skin-support system that incorporates a Velcro-type fastening. You apply a special adhesive-backed strip to the skin on your chest, then line up the corresponding fabric fasteners on the back of the prosthesis with the strips on your chest and press the prosthesis in place. The skin-support strip lasts a week or so, even during swimming, bathing, and showering. You may remove the prosthesis at night, or sleep with it on. According to a study published in 2001 in the journal *Cancer Nursing*, 59.3 percent of the women surveyed preferred the self-adhesive prosthesis over the conventional type, primarily because it seemed to feel more like a part of their body. However, some women preferred the no-muss-no-fuss application of the traditional type, and some complained that the adhesive irritated their skin. Here's what one wearer has to say:

> My first prosthesis was okay because I didn't know any better. But it felt like a plastic thing; it was uncomfortable, although at the time I was grateful for it. My next was much more lifelike and comfortable. But then, when I had my second mastectomy and it was time to get another prosthesis, I discovered "Velcro tits." They had just gotten this new product in the shop and I said, "Let me try it on." I liked the fact that you could wear them either in a bra or without one. I really forget I have them on. I love them! They look and feel so natural that my boyfriend at the time felt them through my blouse and got turned on.

As the study suggests, the main drawback to adhesives is the possibility of an allergic reaction. Although the adhesives are safe for most women, it is wise to do a skin test first, using the liquid adhesive or a small sample of the tape, to detect individual sensitivity. It is best to do the test on the skin of the mastectomy site, especially if you have had radiation, because the skin may be more sensitive there.

## Custom-Made Prostheses

Some stores and private services provide custom-made prostheses. The process involves making a mold of the woman's chest and remaining breast after mastectomy. In some cases they make a mold of the breast before the mastectomy to get a more perfect match. The mold is used to make a prosthesis that more closely matches the shape, weight, and coloring of the missing breast than a mass-produced prosthesis would provide, and that fits the mastectomy site, which will have its own hills and valleys.

A representative of a custom-prosthesis service says, "Most women who come to us are not happy with a standard prosthesis. With this technology, they feel much better. It looks better, it fits better—it locks into their chest like the piece of a puzzle." With this process, you can order a breast that is firm and is worn in a bra, or one that duplicates a natural droop and allows you to go braless if you use adhesive.

Custom-made breast prostheses have been around for quite some time, but the earlier versions had technical problems and never caught on. The process does take time and several visits to complete, and the cost is quite high—up to two thousand dollars. However, insurance companies do partially cover them, and the technology has recently been improved, so this option may become more available and more popular. It offers a reasonable compromise between hit-and-miss mass-produced prostheses and surgical reconstruction, especially if you use adhesive to attach it to the skin.

## Getting the Right Prosthesis for You

The National Cancer Institute offers these tips for prosthesis shoppers:

- ◆ Try on several prostheses to compare the way they feel and look.

- ◆ The prosthesis should feel comfortable and stay in place while you stretch, bend over, and reach.

- ◆ Wear a snug sweater when trying on a prosthesis so you can clearly compare its appearance with your natural breast. Check to see that the top and sides match, and that the nipple, if any, is on the same level as your own and an equal distance from your midline.

- ◆ If the shape and size seem fine, but it feels too light or too heavy, try on another brand or a different weight.

- ◆ Take your time to make sure the prosthesis is comfortable and fits you well.

- ◆ Get a written prescription for a prosthesis from your physician to help ensure payment from your insurance company.

◆ Ask how long the warranty extends and how to take care of the prosthesis.

## Surgical Alternatives to Reconstruction

If you have had a mastectomy or extensive lumpectomy, you may have the option of choosing a surgical procedure that avoids using implants. The tissue-transfer surgeries described in Chapter 3 involve taking muscle and skin from another place on the body and moving them to the site of the mastectomy. (These procedures are also used to create enough skin to accept an implant.) Some women have enough extra fat and tissue in their backs or abdomens to form a natural implant made from their own bodies. Although this is major surgery, some women feel more comfortable knowing their new breast is made from natural material.

Many plastic surgeons are ardent advocates of these flap procedures; others are more cautious. They warn patients that the surgeries often do not work out as well as we would like—the transferred skin is the wrong color and the wrong texture; the new breast tissue is the wrong shape; the flap tissue can die, leaving you worse off than before; and you can be left with cut nerves and weakened muscles in your shoulder or abdomen. As one woman said to me, "I didn't realize I was getting a natural-looking breast in exchange for not being able to get up out of a chair."

Dr. Edward Knowlton argues that "we have to define all risk—not just perceived risk of what a gel implant might cause. You need to look at the mortality rate of a TRAM flap, including higher rates of pulmonary embolism [blood clots that travel to the lungs from the legs and pelvis]. I do these procedures only when others are not feasible." So, although the flap procedures may be worthwhile alternatives to implants for some women, they may be best reserved for women for whom reconstruction is only possible when a flap procedure is used to create a pocket for the implant. However, Dr. Diana Zuckerman feels that combining tissue transfer with implants is "the worst of both worlds."

## Alternatives to Augmentation

When I asked a plastic surgeon about alternatives to augmentation, he laughed and said, "Alternatives? What alternatives? Transsexual surgery? Women come to me and they just want bigger breasts." If you want bigger breasts, implants are the only way to achieve them. (Although there was a report of a woman who increased her bra size from a 34A to a 34C after ten acupuncture treatments!) But if you are unsure about implants, there are three alternatives to consider (they are similar to those available for reconstruction): learning to live with smaller breasts; pads; and uplift surgery. A fourth alternative, fat transfer, is highly controversial.

### The Illusion of Bigger Breasts

There are no physical alternatives to implants that will result in bigger breasts. Despite what many ads claim, there are no creams, massage techniques, devices, or exercises that actually increase the size of breasts. Breast size is determined mostly by genetics, and partly by your overall weight and percentage of body fat. Exercise can improve your posture, which may improve your appearance overall. And it can increase the size and tone of the surrounding muscles that support fatty breast tissue. Along the same lines, you may figure out the types of clothing that look best on you, and that perhaps deemphasize the smallness of your breasts. An image consultant can help devise practical ways to deal with a perceived inadequacy.

Another alternative to surgical augmentation is what used to be called "falsies." Today they're known as push-up pads or contour pads. They used to be made of foam rubber or fluffy polyester, but today they can also be made of the same silicone material that prostheses are made of, for a more natural look and feel. In show biz, actresses who wear them when they play certain roles dub them "chicken cutlets" because of their translucent, meaty look and feel.

You can buy push-up pads in many places where bras are sold—including catalogs and online suppliers. As with breast prostheses to replace a breast, pads only give the illusion of bigger breasts in clothing. When the clothes come off, your breasts will still be small and you must still face that moment of reckoning.

## A Surgical Alternative

A surgical option exists if your goal is to correct sagging breasts. Some women get implants because they lift and firm the breasts somewhat with minimal scarring. However, if you are truly bothered by drooping breasts and want to stay away from surgical implants, you might consider another form of plastic surgery: an "uplift." Although this is still major surgery and creates more visible scars than implantation, it avoids using implants for the sole purpose of achieving a firmer look. The surgical flap procedures used in reconstruction are not used for augmentation purposes.

## A Change in Attitude

Another option is to leave your breasts as they are. But rather than suffering in silence, you may be able to truly break free of our society's emphasis on large breasts. Unlike one-breastedness, small breasts are an anatomical variation, not a physical deformity, even though the condition has its own name: micromastia.

Did you ever consider that "small is beautiful" and small breasts are actually more practical than larger ones? Some of the benefits of smaller breast size are: They don't restrict movement and athletic activity the way large breasts can; their owner can easily lie/sleep on her stomach; they allow their owner to wear skimpy, clingy clothes, and/or to go braless easily; they fit in with the modern aesthetic that values an athletic appearance; they are naturally more perky and less droopy than large breasts, both in a woman's youth and, especially, as she ages; they don't cause back/neck/shoulder aches the way large breasts can.  In addition, you might decide to subscribe to Jane Sprague Zones's view, which sees augmentation as an example of the quick-fix mentality. Zones, a member of the National Women's Health Collective, writes, "The cosmetic surgeon's self-assigned appellation, 'psychiatrist with a knife,' summarizes the perspective that emotional and social benefits may be accrued quickly," without the use of common modalities such as counseling or social change.

You might say "Right on!" to an essay by Barbara Ehrenreich that was published in *Time* magazine. In it she takes some well-aimed, tongue-in-cheek potshots at the way our society makes such a big thing out of small breasts. She writes, "Everyone's life is touched by the tragedy of micromastia because everyone has a friend, sister, co-worker or wife who falls pitifully short in the mammary department. In the past, small groups of health-conscious males, typically gathered at construction sites, would offer free diagnoses to women passersby...." And isn't it ironic that so many women with very large breasts are having them surgically reduced? In fact, almost half as many women have breast reduction sugery every eyar as have augmentation. According to Dr. Diana Zuckerman, many of these women are quoted as saying that they are much less self-consious and more comfortable talking to men who are now able to look them in the eyes when they talk.

You may decide to join the ranks of women who have decided to take the noncosmetic route to feeling attractive and increasing self-esteem. Instead of changing your breast size, you could work on changing your attitude. This might include finding a partner who doesn't require you to have large breasts to be turned on sexually; it might incorporate psychotherapy to help resolve self-image issues to the point where you feel comfortable, desirable, sexy, and self-confident with small breasts.

And you might want to pay attention to a study published in 1992 showing that women greatly overestimate society's taste in breast size. The study involved 130 men and women from seventeen to twenty-five years old who looked at a continuum of figure drawings of women that gradually increased in breast size. When asked which figure they thought the average man or woman would choose, most subjects believed that the very large breasted woman would be the favorite. When they were asked which figure they actually preferred themselves, most indicated that their ideal figure was a good deal smaller, but still somewhat larger than average. So, as J. Kevin Thompson, the author of the study, told the

*New York Times*, "[W]hat we believe society sets as its ideal is way out of line with reality." A plastic surgeon remarked that the new finding might lead some women to reconsider implants. "The notion that men like big breasts is so ingrained in women in our society," he said. "And if a large breast size was perceived of as less desirable or less important, there would be less motivation to change it." He continued that it is sometimes hard to separate our internal drives from the value we place on what everyone else thinks.

Interestingly, the study also found that men overestimate (but to a lesser degree) the chest size that women prefer in men. Other studies have found that women believe men like them thinner than they actually do, creating "an impossible situation" according to Dr. Thompson. "Barbie is an impossible ideal." He hopes the results of his survey might "make women happier with their current size and deter them from something radical such as having an implant." Or you might consider the professional stature, attractiveness, and sex appeal of such modestly endowed celebrities as Kate Moss, Gwyneth Paltrow, Calista Flockhart, Julia Roberts, and Meg Ryan— each of whom, unlike many other actresses, seem to believe they are fine just the way they are.

# Should You Have
# Implants?

Making the decision to have breast reconstruction or augmentation has always been a major step in a woman's life. Today it is more difficult than ever. How do you balance the uncertainty about the long-term safety of implants and the known risks and disadvantages with the potential psychological benefits of implants, especially after mastectomy? If you belong to one of the recently expanded groups of women who qualify for silicone-gel implants, how do you choose between silicone and saline? Today, silicone-gel implants are available for women who want reconstruction after breast cancer surgery, to correct breast asymmetry or deformity, in conjunction with a mastopexy (breast lift), and to replace implants that have been removed. Although silicone-gel implants have still not been "approved" by the FDA, they are available to many more women than when the FDA made its original ruling in 1992. That's because the recently expanded group includes women who are having breast augmentation for the first time and agree to enter a clinical trial, and any woman who has had any type of implant—saline or silicone—and is having it replaced for any reason. This means that although most women may get saline-filled implants the first time around, for their second surgery they may have silicone-gel-filled implants if they wish. Dr. Neal Handel says, "In my practice, the commonest reason for a gel implant is implant replacement." In fact, he says he is now using many more silicone-gel implants than saline. He continues:

> In anyone who has had an implant and needs a replacement, if we feel that a silicone-gel implant will work better, we are allowed to use it. In most of these patients, a gel implant will work better because the tissues have thinned out, and silicone just feels more natural than saline, particularly in someone with a thin layer of breast tissue to hide the implant.

## Steps Toward Making Your Decision

Fortunately, there are some guidelines for you to follow as you take an active role in making your decision.

### 1. Choose the right surgeon.

This is the most important step—not only because the surgeon's technical expertise can greatly influence the results, but also because he or she is in the position of guiding you in making your decision.

- ◆ Get recommendations for several physicians who are board certified in plastic surgery, and get different opinions. Richard Jobe, a plastic surgeon, finds that women who have breast cancer are particularly vulnerable to suggestion and usually do whatever the doctor recommends. "Some surgeons present it as a toggle menu with one procedure automatically following the other—implant, nipple reconstruction, surgery on the opposite breast to improve symmetry," he says. "I look at the process as more of an a la carte menu. None of the follow-up procedures is absolutely necessary."

- ◆ Ask the surgeons how many breast reconstructions or augmentations they have performed in the last year, particularly of the type you are considering, and how long they have been doing breast surgery. The better and more experienced the surgeon, the better your chances of reducing the risk of complications and getting good cosmetic results. Find out the most common complication that he or she experiences with breast implantation, and find out his or her reoperation rate.

◆ Look at before-and-after photographs of the surgeon's work. Make sure you see women who have had the same type of surgery you had or will have, with similar results and similar breast size and shape. Ask to see photos of both the best results and the worst results and make sure the surgeon you are considering did the surgery on these patients. There are plenty of sources for before-and-after breast-implant photos on the web, so you can get a general idea of what to expect. But you need to see the work of the person who will be operating on *your* body.

◆ Choose a plastic surgeon you like, one you feel comfortable with and confident about. I interviewed three plastic surgeons: The first one I just didn't like, the second was gung ho on a latissimus dorsi flap procedure, and the third was just what I was looking for. Not only did we get along, but I also trusted her skills. In addition to the before-and-after photos of her patients, she showed me photos of her oil paintings. She was a true artist—and I certainly felt I deserved to have an artist work on my body. Perhaps not coincidentally, when I had my implant removed and exchanged for saline, I chose a surgeon who was a sculptor.

I can't emphasize this last point strongly enough: The picture is so cloudy right now, with so many conflicting views, that even if you are "well informed" it can be excruciating to make the actual decision, particularly if you are considering reconstruction. While still reeling from a diagnosis of cancer, you may be pressured into deciding whether or not to have immediate reconstruction—a decision that by definition is irrevocable. Susan Leigh, an oncology nurse diagnosed with breast cancer around the time the silicone controversy erupted, found herself paralyzed with indecision. She realized that what was missing was a plastic surgeon she liked and respected and for whom the feeling was mutual. She writes in an article for *Innovations in Oncology Nursing*, "I wanted someone who could help me sort out all the options and conflicting opinions without judgment and sarcasm and could help me make the right decision for me as an individual." She says the only surgeon available to her through her funding source was arrogant and had verbally assaulted her; he rabidly defended silicone-gel implants and then attacked her for seeking information and challenging his opinions. She chose to pay "out of pocket" for a plastic surgeon who was "not only technically and artistically skilled, but was kind, compassionate, a good listener, and appreciated my questions and concerns."

## 2. *Make an informed decision.*

Although it is certainly true that we don't know enough about the safety of implants for any woman to make a truly informed decision, you should at least avail yourself of the information we do have and acquaint yourself with the questions for which we still don't have answers.

- ◆ Read through the chapters in this book about the risks of silicone and saline.

- ◆ Go online and read the stories about women who have implants and have gotten sick.

- ◆ Get the informational material that comes with the implants you are considering, and read the information in the consent form carefully. You will need to get the package insert from your surgeon before the surgery, and from a previous surgery he or she has performed. That's because the insert is sealed in the package, which cannot be opened before the actual surgery without contaminating the implant.

- ◆ Weigh the possible risks against the benefits of both the procedure in general and of silicone versus saline. Although some implants have stayed intact for over twenty years, no one knows the likely lifespan in any individual case. Realize that implants are not designed to last a lifetime—you will probably need to have them replaced at some point, and most likely every eight to ten years. One manufacturer likens this to "many other plastic surgery procedures which are commonly repeated to maintain patient satisfaction." The difference here is we are talking about health and well-being, not psychological satisfaction.

◆ Think twice about augmentation if you are at high risk for future breast cancer because of family history, premalignant breast changes, or previous breast cancer. You may decide the benefits are not worth the risk of an obstructed mammogram missing the early signs of breast cancer, of the implant increasing your risk of breast cancer, or of the possibility of further deranging your immune system if you have had chemotherapy.

◆ Get counseling if autoimmune disease runs in your family. This can be as simple as talking over your family health history with your physician. In addition, you may want to explore certain laboratory tests that indicate if you might be prone to developing lupus or scleroderma. These include antinuclear antibody titer (ANA), rheumatoid factor, and sedimentation rate. Dr. Edward Knowlton feels that "even if there is only the tiniest evidence of a relationship in people who are genetically predisposed, a gel implant should be avoided." The patient-information brochures from implant manufacturers McGhan and Mentor both warn that "safety and effectiveness has not been established" in women with "autoimmune diseases such as lupus and scleroderma, conditions that interfere with wound healing and blood clotting, a weakened immune system," or "reduced blood supply to the breast tissue."

◆ Discuss your concerns and wishes with your plastic surgeon, and ask him or her to explain anything you don't understand. Ask how many reoperations you can expect to have during your lifetime, how your breast(s) will look if you choose to have the implant(s) removed without replacing them, how you can expect your implanted breast(s) to look as you get older, and what would be your options if you are dissatisfied with the results of your implant(s).

◆ Take your time deciding. Unless you are considering immediate reconstruction (see "Timing for Reconstruction," starting on page 187), there is no reason to hurry a decision.

## 3. *Know why you want implants.*

◆ Talk to or meet with women who have made a variety of decisions. How and why did they choose? Are they satisfied with the results? Would they do it again?

◆ Do it for yourself, not to please others. Doing it for another person is the worst reason to have implant surgery. Talk about augmentation or reconstruction with your partner. My husband made it clear he wasn't bothered by my lopsidedness. In fact, he was more afraid of the additional surgery than I was. I had to reassure him I was doing it for myself, not because of him, and that I felt the surgery would make me feel better.

◆ Have realistic expectations—especially if your implant is for reconstruction—about both the physical results and the psychological and social changes. Your confidence and self-image may improve, your sex life may pick up or be restored, or it may not. Having surgery will not solve all your problems.

Loren Eskenazi, a plastic surgeon who specializes in breast surgery, offers this advice:

You need to be very well informed, shop around, and think about it. For women who are flat chested, implants are still an incredible boon to their lives. For those who are not really flat chested, who are just doing it for a larger cup size, they need to think twice. This whole controversy reminds us that the decision to change one's body is not to be taken lightly in any respect. This is true whether it takes an hour and is cheap, or takes ten hours and is expensive.

## Reducing Risks

Most preventive efforts are focused on reducing capsular contracture. This is not only the most common adverse effect; it can also increase the risk of other adverse effects. As of now, there are no surefire ways of preventing it, nor of predicting who is most likely to experience it. However, you and your plastic surgeon can take steps that may reduce the chances of its occurring. None of these approaches is guaranteed, and there is considerable debate as to their effectiveness, so if you elect to have implants you should discuss the merits of the various options with your surgeon.

### Type and Texture of Implant

Many plastic surgeons have found that using saline implants reduces the likelihood of contracture. Perhaps it is because a saline implant inherently avoids the silicone-gel bleed that may be a major factor in causing the capsule to contract. However, other surgeons have found no difference in this respect. In addition, many surgeons have found that using implants with a textured silicone shell markedly reduces contracture, but again, other surgeons have found the opposite to be true. Neal Handel and colleagues conducted a large study, published in 1995, that found texture made no difference in the contracture rate. "What we did find was that texturing greatly increases risk of palpability, rippling, and waviness of implants—particularly if they are saline and placed above the muscle. The texturing grips the surface of the tissue, like the traction of sneakers on a wet surface," Dr. Handel says. "That's why most people have reverted back to smooth implants."

## Placement of Implant

In reconstruction, the implant generally goes beneath the pectoralis (chest) muscle, because there is not enough tissue available otherwise. However, there is an option in augmentation, and Dr. Paul Striker feels that positioning of the implant above or beneath the muscle is a "hotly debated issue" that will never be completely resolved. Many surgeons find that putting the implant beneath the chest muscle helps reduce encapsulization, perhaps because the pressure from the chest muscle keeps the scar tissue from shrinking and hardening. However, in Neal Handel's 1995 study, placement of the implant above or below the muscle did not make a difference in the rate of contracture.

But there are other factors to consider in placement. Placing the implant beneath the muscle also means it is less likely to obscure a mammogram that could detect breast cancer in its early stages. Handel says that almost all the studies done to date suggest that implants positioned under the pectoralis muscle interfere the least with mammography. He believes this should be taken into account, especially in women who are in their late thirties and forties—when the risk of breast cancer begins to rise. Another consideration, however, is that placing an implant under the muscle requires a more extensive operation than placing the implant above the muscle, with greater surgical risks and longer recovery time. Other factors, having to do with aesthetics, are discussed below.

## Surgical Technique

Your surgeon needs to create a large enough pocket for the implant. If the pocket is too small, contracture is more likely. In addition, excess or uncontrolled bleeding from the surgery contributes to capsular contracture. So, the more meticulous the surgeon is about controlling bleeding, the less blood there is to create infection and inflammatory response, which increases scar tissue.

Putting in a drain after surgery may reduce the incidence of hematomas and seromas (blood and fluid accumulation, respectively), which could later cause contractures. And since there have been concerns voiced over the increased risk of saline implants becoming infected, techniques to reduce this possibility are also a consideration. Although Dr. Eskenazi has never seen it occur, she says the theory is that the fluid could become contaminated when the implant is filled during surgery, so due care must be taken during this process. Dr. Striker says, "Organisms don't really grow in sterile saline, and although the silicone shell is permeable—fluids go in and fluids go out—bacteria are too large to penetrate." Eskenazi acknowledges that a low-grade bacterial or fungal infection around the implant is a possibility. She says, "A lot of the textured implants cause the body to produce a fluid around them, caused by the constant rubbing of the implant against the capsule. That fluid can 'seed' bacteria that are normally present in the bloodstream," and not necessarily introduced during the surgery.

## Massage and Exercise

Some surgeons teach patients to massage their implants after surgery as a further step toward possibly reducing encapsulization, but lately manufacturers and others have been warning that this may increase the chance of a rupture. Striker, for one, says this newer concern is nonsense; he continues to give his patients specific instructions for a type of self-massage using compression exercises that keep the capsule expanded. Although at first it was very painful to do so, my surgeon recommended that I massage the implant after I had reached a certain stage of healing. Elizabeth Morgan, author of *The Complete Book of Plastic Surgery*, puts the implant between the breast and the muscle and then advises her patients to do specific types of exercises for at least six months after surgery. After six months, the scar tissue loses its "shrinkability." At that point she recommends resistance-type exercises that keep the chest muscles stretched, such as using Nautilus machines, rowing machines, arm weights, or swimming. However, these are all individual recommendations, and there are no studies on the advisability of massage or exercise that I am aware of.

## Other Measures

As a further safeguard against bleeding, it is wise to avoid taking aspirin for two weeks before and after surgery. Some surgeons recommend that women avoid scheduling surgery near or during their menstrual period, because the blood's clotting ability is altered. Striker advises his patients to stop smoking before surgery to encourage healing. To reduce scar formation, he also prescribes vitamin E supplements to be taken twice a day, beginning one day before surgery and continuing for as long as the implants are in place.

To stop formation of scar tissue, some surgeons have administered steroids, either orally or put directly around the implant. However, these hormones have several undesirable side effects: They increase the chance of infection; interfere with healing; may cause larger, redder scar formation; and can cause the breasts to weaken and droop.

## Aesthetics

Obviously, you want your implants to be as aesthetically pleasing as possible—to have a natural-looking shape and feel, to be soft, to be ripple-free, and to stay in a natural-looking position. Since contracture looks unnatural, many of the factors that affect contracture play into the aesthetic of implants. But let's begin with the most obvious factor—the shape and size of the implant itself.

Implants come in different shapes and sizes. They can be "rounded"—a half-dome shape—or "shaped" or "contoured"—resembling a half-teardrop shape. The rounded style may produce a more rounded appearance to the upper breast, and the shaped style can provide a more gently downward-sloping contour. Dr. Eskenazi says, "Shaped saline implants do not always give the most natural appearance. They can rotate, and when a woman lies on her back, they do not fall off the chest wall to the side," as a natural breast would. She continues, "It is possible to get a natural breast shape using a round implant. It has to do with the way the skin envelope is dissected at the time of surgery."

Size is a factor—if you want a breast implant that is too large for your frame, you will look out of proportion. If you choose one that is too large for the amount of tissue you have, you may be able to see or feel the implant's edges, and your breasts may droop excessively over time. But if you choose one that is too small, you may be unhappy with the result. Dr. Striker says he has never had a patient complain that her augmented breasts were too large—but he has had patients who were disappointed that they did not go larger.

The material used is also a factor in aesthetics and overall final appearance. No matter what shape implant you put in, a strong contracture will convert it to a round shape—as the capsule gets tighter and tighter, you get a rounder and rounder ball.

Eskenazi is one of those plastic surgeons who feels that saline does not look or feel as natural as silicone gel. "It's a bag of water," she says. "Those who say it looks fine—well, what's fine? What some people consider fine or okay I wouldn't consider acceptable." However, she also says:

> A soft implant, be it saline or silicone, is always more natural than an encapsulated hard one. Thus, I prefer saline since it has a lower rate of encapsulization than silicone. If rippling becomes a problem over time, we can always switch the woman over to silicone gel. In my practice, very few women do this for augmentation—the rate of switching to silicone gel is higher for reconstruction because the overlying skin is thinner and the ripples are more obvious.

As a final word, Eskenazi concludes, "After trying all the different types of implants made, I have come full circle to smooth saline implants, either above or below the muscle."

Paul Striker, who used saline exclusively long before the FDA restrictions, says:

> I've seen really good saline and silicone implants—you can't tell the difference. I've seen bad examples of both, too. I think the incidence of good is greater with salt water. Sure you're going to get some wrinkling, and textured implants

you tend to feel a bit more because the shell is thicker and
you can sometimes feel the edges. But there's a softer breast.
So you have to ask yourself which you prefer: A softer breast
but one where you can feel the implant a bit? Or a firmer
breast where you can't feel the implant edge?

Where your surgeon places the implant—above or below the
pectoralis muscle—can also make a big difference in the aesthetic
results. Factors to consider are the amount of breast tissue you
have (the more you have, the less obvious the implant), the implant
filler (saline sloshes and wrinkles), the amount of natural droop
(the more you have, the more obvious the implant), and your
degree of physical activity and muscle tone (a submuscular implant
gets compressed and deformed when you flex the muscle).

Dr. Handel finds that placing the implant submuscularly gets
the best aesthetic results if:

- ◆ you have very little breast tissue

- ◆ you are using a saline implant

- ◆ your breast is not very droopy

- ◆ you are not very physically active

Placing it above the muscle is more aesthetically pleasing if:

- ◆ you have an adequate amount of breast tissue

- ◆ you are using silicone gel

- ◆ your breast is quite droopy

- ◆ you are physically active

Another consideration in submuscular placement is the likelihood of greater problems if the implant leaks or ruptures, because
the silicone may damage the muscle and also be harder to remove.
Dr. Eskenazi cautions that there are no hard and fast rules as to
the positioning of the implant:

The factors are variable from patient to patient. What does the patient want? What does she do? What type of aesthetic does she like? What type of chest wall does she have? How much fat does she have; how much breast tissue? If you have a very muscular girl who jumps around and does a lot of aerobics and doesn't mind a round-looking breast, I'd go over the muscle with saline. If you have someone who doesn't do a lot of exercise and wants a more natural appearance, I'd put saline under the muscle.

## Silicone Gel from Abroad?

Because of the FDA restrictions, most American women cannot get silicone-gel implants legally outside of a clinical trial. A trial entails paperwork, regular checkups, and lab tests for years following surgery. So a growing number of women are looking elsewhere: Silicone-gel implants are still available in almost every other country (except Canada, Taiwan, and Australia). At one time, the most popular locations for obtaining silicone implants were in the Caribbean, Mexico, South America, and Europe. More recently, Thailand has become all the rage. Perhaps, since the FDA has expanded the group of women for whom silicone is available, we will see a slowing of this ridiculous development. Such "implants a-go-go" leave you little recourse if something goes wrong. Once you leave the hospital (or surgical condo) where the surgery is performed, there is little or no follow-up care. American doctors in port cities are being asked to treat implant-related problems—poor results, infection, bleeding, and older types of implants that are more bleed- and rupture-prone—in women whom they have never seen before.

As Dr. Striker observes, "It's a bad idea. You are thousands of miles away from your doctor. You are in a strange country. If you have a complication, you can't go back to the doctor that easily. He may not even be there anymore! And who knows what they actually inserted?"

## Reducing Risks in Reconstruction

Women who have undergone mastectomy face the additional problem of having too little tissue to work with, which adds to the risk of contracture. Tissue expanders help relieve this problem, as do flap procedures, but there are limitations and problems with both of these. Edward Knowlton, a plastic surgeon who specializes in reconstruction, says it is most important to maintain as much skin and muscle as possible. "For this, you need to work with your general surgeon before the mastectomy." Fortunately, he says, we are undergoing a "revolution in mastectomy," in which surgeons are taking less skin and muscle than in the past. He believes there is even more hope for the future. For example, he has developed a procedure that involves cutting away only the nipple-areola complex and removing the breast tissue through the relatively small hole made in the skin. He then creates a mini latissimus dorsi flap of skin and some muscle to replace the areola and expand the pectoralis muscle. "This," he says, "preserves the skin of the breast and avoids creating an extensive submuscular pocket for the implant. You also don't need to perform an uplift on the opposite breast to achieve symmetry."

Twenty years ago, when my surgeon was preparing me for my implant surgery, she advised me to start taking eight hundred units of vitamin E every day. She showed me how to do compression massage on my reconstructed breast. Although no one told me to, I resumed my regular exercise program shortly after my surgery. In addition, I had a double-lumen implant, with saline on the outside. Perhaps one or some combination of these strategies worked, because although I did not have a tissue expander or flap surgery, I had minimal capsular contracture. My reconstructed breast was firmer than my natural breast, but it certainly wasn't hard; it had a relatively natural shape, and it hadn't moved up to a higher position on my chest. However, I must say that the results of my second reconstruction are even better than the first. Again, there may be multiple reasons for this—the skin and muscle were already stretched from the first implant, the second implant was smooth saline, and I wore a surgical drain and a compression bandage after the surgery. Even my oncologist—who has seen many reconstructed breasts—was extremely pleased with the results.

## Timing for Reconstruction

Reconstruction can be done anytime after a mastectomy—one, five, ten, or thirty years later. And age is no barrier. There are seventy-year-old women who have had reconstruction. An increasing number of women are choosing immediate reconstruction—in other words, at the time of the mastectomy. You may find this is the best time for you, too.

Immediate reconstruction offers several advantages. It helps reduce the emotional anguish caused by losing a breast following the devastating news of a diagnosis of breast cancer. Since it avoids a second surgery in addition to the mastectomy, it can reduce the time spent under anesthesia, the time spent in the hospital, and the patient's discomfort. On the downside, the cosmetic results may not be as good as if the surgery is done at a later date. There may also be an increased risk of complications such as infection, bleeding, and hardening around the implant.

A reconstructed breast is never perfect, never exactly like the natural breast that was removed. Therefore some argue that women who undergo immediate reconstruction are more apt to be disappointed with the results. They compare the stitched-together, nippleless mound with the breast that used to be there, rather than with the flat nothingness they would have lived with if they had delayed reconstruction. Most plastic surgeons and women feel this is nonsense, on a par with those who suggest women should delay reconstruction because they should fully mourn the loss of their breast.

Some studies support the value of immediate reconstruction. Wendy Schain, Ed.D., and David Wellisch, Ph.D., studied women with immediate and delayed reconstruction. Both groups were equally satisfied with the results. But the women who delayed the procedure were more depressed, anxious, hostile, and emotionally distressed. Another study, by Laurie Stevens, found women who opted for immediate reconstruction were better able to integrate the new breast, to feel it was their own—not just a mound stuck on their chest. She, too, found these women to be less depressed and anxious; they maintained sexual functioning and desire and had fewer feelings of low self-esteem or diminished femininity. However, more recent research indicates that reconstruction in general is not the booster it is cracked up to be. A review paper by Diana Harcourt published in 2000 undertook a thorough search of the existing literature examining breast reconstruction in terms of relevant psychological constructs, especially in relation to coping and decision-making. Harcourt writes that she found "methodological flaws with much of the existing research in this area, in particular the reliance upon retrospective designs and the inappropriate use of randomized controlled trials." She concluded that "existing research into the psychological aspects of breast reconstruction is limited" and that "more methodologically rigorous research is needed." A study published in 2000 by the National Cancer Institute found that women with breast cancer who were treated with a mastectomy or mastectomy plus reconstruction responded similarly on a questionnaire that measured health-related quality of life, body image, and physical and sexual functioning.

It is probably unwise to have immediate reconstruction if you are at all unsure about whether it is the right thing for you. In this case, go ahead with the mastectomy and make your decision about reconstruction later, when you are ready to deal with it. Sometimes making yet another decision is too much to handle after all the other treatment decisions you face.

Dr. Richard Jobe is not enthusiastic about immediate reconstruction. He explains why:

> I have talked to many women about reconstruction before they had their mastectomies. It was my observation that there was very little correlation between what the patient thought she wanted at the time and what she finally did. Some patients said they didn't want it, but ultimately did,

and vice versa. Patients on the verge of having a mastectomy really aren't in a position to make a definitive decision as to whether they need and want reconstruction.

Dr. Loren Eskenazi thinks that every woman who is not having a breast-conserving procedure (lumpectomy) should at least be offered immediate reconstruction. In addition to subjecting women to one surgery and one general anesthesia as opposed to two, while only adding another hour or so to the surgery, she believes the results are better. She says:

> You can do what's called a skin-sparing mastectomy, which leaves you enough skin to form a fold so you have a normal, ptotic [drooping] breast. You can't do that with delayed reconstruction, because the plastic surgeon marks the surgical area for the cancer surgeon. This means that the cancer surgeon and the plastic surgeon have to work together. That should not be a problem in this day and age.

Together with photographer Terry Lorant, Dr. Eskenazi has published a book called *Reconstructing Aphrodite*. Published in 2001, it shows beautiful photographs of women with immediate and delayed reconstruction, and describes the process in detail.

I have met women who have had good and bad experiences with immediate reconstruction. Here are the comments of two of them:

◆ I was thrilled to wake up after surgery knowing I had a breast. It made the diagnosis seem not quite so bad. Although I did have to have the surgery redone at a later date, at least at the time I didn't have to adjust to losing a breast in addition to the diagnosis of cancer and the side effects of chemotherapy.

◆ I realized I had made a mistake in having immediate reconstruction. Not that I wouldn't have had it ultimately, but I did have an implant-related infection at one point, which I didn't need on top of the chemo, let me tell you. And the other thing was, I resented that I had locked myself into that decision. What if I felt strongly that I didn't want an implant afterward? I was worried about the adverse effects of silicone, so I ended up with saline—and that was another decision I just didn't feel ready to deal with.

## Timing for Augmentation

Recently, there has been a surge of interest in cosmetic surgery of all types among young people. Although some surgeries may be appropriate, augmentation is not recommended for young girls. It is best to wait until the breasts have reached their full development—usually at about eighteen years of age. Some would argue that even eighteen is too young, and a woman should wait until she is in her twenties. Physical maturity is only one side of the coin—a certain amount of emotional maturity is needed, too. Diana Zuckerman, Ph.D., points out that most women gain weight in their late teens and early twenties, and as a result, their breasts will naturally increase in size. In addition, an eighteen-year-old woman who wants to look like the latest voluptuous (and probably augmented) teen idol may change her mind when she is a bit older. The decision to have breast implants is a lifetime decision; with the way our technology currently stands, a woman who has implants at the age of eighteen and lives to the age of eighty faces the prospect of at least seven more surgeries to replace them—and possibly more, if she has complications. If she decides at some point to have her implants removed and not replaced, she may end up with less breast tissue than she started out with or distorted and scarred breasts, not to mention difficulty breastfeeding or systemic disease.

Some recommend delaying implant surgery until after a woman is through with childbearing. The reason is twofold: There are unanswered questions about the effects of silicone on a fetus or nursing child, and a possibility exists that pregnancy and breast-feeding will change the shape of the breasts and affect the results of the augmentation.

The American College of Radiology recommends that a woman have a mammogram if she is over thirty-five and plans to undergo breast augmentation. A mammogram will detect suspicious lumps beforehand and serve as a baseline against which she and her physicians can compare future mammograms.

## Who Pays?

Implants for augmentation are considered cosmetic, and costs are not reimbursed by insurance companies. Insurance companies are required by law to cover breast reconstruction, but not all of them include nipple reconstruction. Be sure to ask how much the surgery will cost; whether your insurance company will pay for the initial surgery as well as subsequent complications; whether you can make installment payments; and whether your surgeon will perform any follow-up procedures at a reduced fee or no fee. With the complete information in hand, you may end up not having surgery—or at least delaying it—and opting for one of the alternatives described in Chapter 7.

# 9

# The Future of Implants: Where Do We Go from Here?

In the previous edition of this book, I wrote, "It would be an understatement to say the future of silicone-gel implants—or of any implant—is uncertain." The future is still uncertain, but today, implants are more popular than ever—between 1997 and 2000, the number of breast-augmentation procedures doubled, and the incidence of reconstruction more than doubled. Saline implants, which still consist of a silicone shell, are now approved by the FDA and available to any woman, despite safety studies that followed women for only three years. And the FDA has also expanded the availability of silicone-gel implants beyond the original group of women eligible after 1992. Women's-health advocates fear that silicone gel will follow in the footsteps of saline and eventually be available to any woman.

## A Better Silicone—or Something Else?

Clearly, silicone as an implant material—either as gel filler or as elastomer shell—is not going away soon. This, in spite of the fact that we still don't know the long-term effects of silicone on the body, and in spite of the fact that what we do know is appalling: There's a high rate of local complications, including painful contracture, hardening, ruptures, and frequent reoperations.

Surely, if we can put a man on the moon, we can come up with safer materials for implants. Well, maybe, maybe not. It is not that easy to find something that will feel natural, be compatible with the body chemistry, and, hopefully, last longer than eight or ten years.

As an example of how difficult it is, remember the implant filled with soybean oil I mentioned earlier in this book? In the early 1990s a company called LipoMatrix began testing an implant called the TRILUCENT. The design grew out of the hard work of a team of plastic surgeons and radiologists from Washington University. The triglyceride filler was very close in composition to human fat, the main component of breast tissue, and thus much more radiolucent than silicone gel or even saline. This would presumably result in a much clearer image during mammography. LipoMatrix's president, Terry Knapp, a plastic surgeon, said his implant had other advantages over existing implants. The shell was stronger, and did not leak filler or shed molecules into the tissues. The oily triglyceride filler was a natural lubricant, which supposedly would prevent abrasion of the shell over time—a cause of leakage. Animal research showed that if the implant did rupture, it would deflate over the course of a few weeks, and the oil would be absorbed, metabolized, and excreted by the body in the same way as dietary triglycerides (vegetable oil). Compared with saline implants, which wore out after 350,000 abrasion test cycles, the TRILUCENT implant was still intact after 10 million cycles. However, as mentioned earlier in this book, the TRILUCENT was a failure. In 1999, the Medical Device Agency (MDA), the British equivalent of the FDA, removed this implant from the market in the United Kingdom because of reports of adverse events. They were concerned that breakdown products of the soybean filler that was removed from some women were significantly different from the breakdown products predicted during preclinical testing. These breakdown products, they feared, might eventually have toxic effects that could cause cancer. In 2000, the MDA issued a Hazard Warning entitled: "TRILUCENT Breast Implants: Recommendation to Remove," that pertained to all TRILUCENT breast implants worldwide. It recommended that women immediately have their implants removed and that they avoid becoming pregnant or breastfeeding until they had their implants removed. The TRILUCENT was never approved by the FDA, except for clinical trials. The FDA developed a plan to contact all the women in the United States who had the implants and requested that they be evaluated and be told of the MDA findings and recommendations. McGhan issued a press release that stated:

> In consultation with the FDA, McGhan Medical wishes to assure patients involved in the U.S. and Canadian TRILUCENT trials that it will provide a comprehensive program of support and assistance for women who have received these breast implants, under which it will cover medical expenses associated with their removal and replacement. McGhan Medical will provide specific information about the program to patients and surgeons involved in these studies.

Other fillers are being tested. One approach attempts to address the low viscosity and unnatural feel inherent in saline implants. Researchers are testing implants filled with polyethylene glycol (PEG) plus saline. The PEG thickens the saline and, according to its proponents, more closely approximates the "feel" of normal breast tissue while preserving the safety of saline. They are also more radiolucent than silicone or plain saline. Another type of implant, made of polyvinylpurolidone (PVP), or hydrogel, was being investigated, but has been taken off the market because of inadequacies in the manufacturers' safety assessments of the hydrogel fillings. Hydrogel is used in contact lenses, medicines, surgical dressings, and food. However, according to Dr. Diana Zuckerman and Rachel Flynn of the National Center for Policy Research (CPR) for Women & Families, it was banned in implants because the FDA found a "lack of long-term toxicity data or clinical follow-up, methodological flaws in some of the pre-clinical tests, and pathological changes in a study of rabbits." They continue:

The removal of these kinds of implants from the market, after they had been enthusiastically praised by doctors and patients, serves as a reminder that the long-term risks of implants are not always obvious during the first few years of use. That is why studies of the risks of long-term use are essential to establish the safety of implants.

Still another approach seeks to make silicone gel safer. A new silicone-gel implant is being tested that has a more cohesive consistency—like solid gelatin—than does the less viscous silicone gel that is currently being used. It does not spill or run even when cut, and, theoretically, it would not bleed or migrate throughout the body.

Dr. Susan Kolb, the Atlanta plastic surgeon who had silicone-gel implants, got sick, and exchanged them for saline, says, "I am truly in the middle of this issue. I see the benefits of implants, and I also see the problems. I can't be totally against implants because I have them in my body." Like me, she wants to keep her implants, and she wants science to take the problems seriously so they can be improved when we need our implants replaced.

"Silicone has to be studied and be made safe," she continues, "because it is the number-one implant material that we have. So far, I don't know of anything that you can make a breast implant out of...or encase a pacemaker in." She believes that silicone gel can't be used safely because "like nuclear waste, there is nothing that can contain it. But as far as the silicone shell—we should be able to figure out how to put that in safely, and then modulate the immune system so it doesn't go berserk." Take one of my personal experiences as an example. When I first got contact lenses, they were rigid, painful devices. Now we have developed contact lenses that are soft and comfortable and still get the job done.

## Silicone Tests

Although recent studies show that silicone does not make most women sick over the short term, studies may yet prove that a certain percentage of women are sensitive to silicone. Studies suggest that there is a genetic marker called histocompatibility complex (HLA) for women who are more susceptible to the kind of poorly defined autoimmune disorders that seem to be triggered by silicone implants, as well as more susceptible to capsular contracture. Tests indicate that some people have a general autoimmune predisposition, and this could lead to testing specifically for silicone sensitivity. Melvin Spira, professor of surgery in the Division of Plastic Surgery at Baylor College of Medicine, in Houston, says:

> It's important that we realize that there may be a subset of patients who are predisposed to these poorly understood and poorly characterized autoimmune phenomena. It may not be a specific disease. It's possible that in the future we may have a skin test that will identify women who are prone to problems with silicone implants and they will not receive an implant.

Also, it would be helpful to have tests that determine whether silicone is present in other parts of the body, as well as whether a woman might be sensitive to it. There are already tests that detect silicone in the blood and urine, but silicone can come from many sources, including medicines and cosmetics, as well as from a silicone implant, so these tests do not really give us useful information. A test for silicone sensitivity would be more valuable, but no such test exists at this time.

Dr. Edward Knowlton says we must start thinking now about patients who actually are at risk, to develop a preoperative, standardized panel of tests to identify the majority of the patients who would be at risk if they received an implant or any other foreign body. He says in the future we also have to learn to more clearly identify patients who enter a doctor's office and are already sick from their implants. Although he feels the incidence is very low, he says:

> We need to identify those who are being pushed over into the disease earlier in life, or whose disease is being made worse. This diagnosis will be one of probability that there is a suspicion that the implant is making people worse. It won't

click in clearly like diabetes, and we will not be able to say cause and effect—but there will be a suspicion that this is going to happen.

Knowlton admits that what he's proposing would be a crapshoot, but with testing "we want to be able to at least file down the edges of the dice as much as we can. We want to...have some assurance that when we make the diagnosis, the patient is going to feel better. Explanting implants for many patients is very difficult emotionally, so we want to be as sure as possible that we're not taking them out unnecessarily."

## Improving the FDA's Role and Responsibility

It's no secret that the FDA could do a better job of insuring our safety. In January 1993, one year after the FDA placed a moratorium on silicone implants, an important report was released, titled *The FDA's Regulation of Silicone Breast Implants*. It was based on a three-year investigation by the Human Resources and Intergovernmental Relations Subcommittee of the House Committee on Government Operations. The report traces the FDA's role in the breast-implant fiasco and concludes that:

◆ Patients were misled about the risks of the implants for more than fifteen years.

◆ Patients continued to be misled under the "urgent need" provision, because the FDA failed to monitor the program properly. For example, informed-consent forms for approximately one-third of the women who underwent surgery were missing from the files; and the consent forms were "watered down" due to pressure from plastic surgeons and the American Medical Association, "thus continuing the FDA's pattern of ignoring evidence of problems because of industry pressure."

◆ The FDA's public statements about breast implants mini-
mized the risk.

◆ Professional pro-implant lobbyists included former FDA officials and provided patient lobbyists with misleading information.

The report also recommended new legislation to close the
revolving door between the FDA and industry—for example, the
hiring of former FDA employees as lobbyists for plastic surgeons
and the implant industry—which creates conflict of interest. The
report concluded that no safeguards were in place to ensure that
physicians or manufacturers comply with FDA policy, and that as
soon as media attention drifted, "it was business as usual at FDA."

Can public pressure encourage the FDA to turn over a new
leaf? Perhaps. As part of its ongoing review of pre-1976 devices,
in 1993 the FDA proposed that manufacturers of testicular implants
submit scientific data showing they are safe and effective, and the
FDA called for data for a number of other devices. An internal
report released in March 1993 characterized safety tests on some
commonly used medical devices as grossly inferior, sometimes using
too few patients to detect possible side effects, and in some cases
so poorly carried out they were "not up to the level of fifth-grade
science," said Bruce Burlington, the new director of the FDA's Center for Devices and Radiologic Health, to *The New York Times*.

Since then, safety data on saline implants have been supplied
by the manufacturers, but the studies followed women for only
three years. What happens to them after three years? We need
studies that include women who have had reconstruction; we need
studies that aim to determine whether silicone causes nonclassic
forms of autoimmune disease, infection, or toxic poisoning; we need
studies that follow a large enough number of women over a long
enough period of time to actually have some meaning for women
living real lives. We need studies honestly designed in a way that
finds out whether implants are safe—not studies cleverly designed
to prove that they are safe. We need studies that are funded and
conducted by impartial researchers—in other words, funded by the

government—and not by plastic surgeons and implant companies who have a vested interest in proving these products are safe.

In November 2001, a Congressional hearing on breast implants took place, held by the Health Subcommittee of the House of Representatives Energy and Commerce Committee. The hearing was held at the request of Rep. Roy Blunt (R-Missouri) and Rep. Gene Green (D-Texas). According to Dr. Diana Zuckerman, this hearing marked "a milestone." It was the first hearing that was sympathetic to health problems linked to implants since the one that resulted from the 1990 investigation of the FDA's regulation of breast implants, which she initiated. The hearing was regarding a piece of legislation known as The Breast Implant Research and Information Act. This bill would insure that women would have the most accurate, recent scientific research available in making their decisions about implants, and would require independent long-term follow-up studies of implants. It would specifically:

- ◆ Require the National Institutes of Health (NIH) to intensify their research into the health implications of breast implants

- ◆ Expand and intensify FDA efforts to disseminate accurate, current data about implants

- ◆ Strengthen FDA postmarket evaluations of saline implants

- ◆ Require the FDA to complete an ongoing criminal investigation of Mentor, a company that was accused of data manipulation in its trials of breast implants

Dr. Zuckerman testified before the Committee as follows:

If Congress doesn't require that these important studies be conducted by NIH, it is unlikely they ever will be....I hope the committee will also undertake a careful review of the FDA regarding the long-term safety data on breast implants. Breast implants have been sold for almost forty years, and yet the FDA had never required long-term safety data.

## Corporate Trust and Accountability

On 19 February 1992, Sidney Wolfe gave testimony before the FDA implant-advisory committee that included harsh words about the companies that make and sell drugs and devices. In the years just preceding his testimony, three major drug companies had withheld data from the FDA, which caused the agency to approve drugs that later were banned because together they killed hundreds of people and injured thousands. Other companies have been or are being investigated for possible criminal behavior. Wolfe said he hoped the manufacturers of silicone implants would join them. He believes we need to strengthen the FDA's authority to subpoena company records and to end gag orders on corporate health and safety data. He feels we also need to develop a healthy "sense of distrust for companies such as those who place their self-indulgent marketing goals above the health of the people."

The 1993 congressional report mentioned above also revealed that in 1992, Dow Corning disclosed that the company had sold implants to doctors before they were shown to be safe in animals, failed to disclose problems with the implants, and submitted fabricated information about quality control. In addition, the report referred to newly available internal memoranda from legal discovery conducted during breast-implant litigation. For example, in 1978 Surgitek executives requested that a study of silicone in dogs be terminated when the dogs were found to have serious illnesses, and demanded that the animals be killed and their organs destroyed. Bristol-Myers Squibb memoranda from the 1970s and 1980s discuss concerns about implant rupture and silicone-gel migration. We also now know that Dow Corning did not make public a 1975 study showing that a purified form of one type of silicone (called D4) used in implants was highly toxic to the immune system of mice. This study evolved out of the fact that the company had two research teams—one of which found that silicone was biologically active, and the other that determined silicone was inert. The company decided to listen to the latter team and halt research into the immunological activity of silicone in 1975.

A lawyer for the plaintiffs in the class-action suit against the implant companies believes this research was the smoking gun that proves Dow Corning was well aware of the immunological effects of certain silicones and that they made a decision based on profits, not safety. Don Bennett, one of the scientists involved in the research, explained to the *New York Times* that one team consisted of chemists and toxicologists, the other of biologists. The notion of silicone's biocompatibility was widely accepted by scientists, and in those heady days it was hoped that artificial body parts would revolutionize medicine. Dow Corning, which was after all a chemical company (remember the ad slogan "Better living through chemistry"?), chose to listen to its chemists, who typically think that biology will take care of itself, according to Bennett.

## Our Implants, Ourselves

The "implant circus" was messy and may not be completely over yet, but perhaps the fracas can teach us some valuable lessons. We need to educate ourselves as consumers, to ask our doctors questions about our personal health, and to have more of a voice when health-policy decisions are made. Dr. Edward Knowlton feels it is crucial that health consumers better understand terms and concepts such as "risk-benefit ratio," "risk and safety," "anecdotal evidence," "coincidental medical conditions," and "cause and effect." Otherwise, we cannot begin to judge for ourselves whether any particular argument has merit or not, nor can we participate in medical debates about implants or any other issue.

Barbara Carter, consultant on the psychosocial effects of cancer, speaks of another educational task before us. We need to realize that most product testing is done by the manufacturers of the drugs or devices in question, and that they have a vested interest in providing evidence that these things are safe. "The consumer needs to know and understand this," she says, "and to look at the motivation of whoever is presenting that information. We need to protect the consumer by having people without this motivation to *do* the research and to *scrutinize* the research, in order to decrease bias."

Then follows the question: Who pays for this objective research? Most of the breast-implant studies have been paid for by manufacturers out of their research-and-development budgets. Do we want to pay for this out of public money? Or should we have the manufacturers put up the money for outside testing, with safeguards to prevent kickbacks? Remember, implant manufacturing is a multibillion dollar business—driven by capitalism, not altruism.

And, finally, we have to remind ourselves that any device, any surgical procedure, will have certain risks. We need to ask: What are *reasonable* risks? What price are we willing to pay in exchange for the benefits? And what are we willing to spend now in time, money, and effort to make sure we get all the information we need to answer these questions?

# Five Important Issues to Explore When Considering Implantation—or Explantation

## by Sharyn Higdon Jones

1.   Be clear on your reasons for having implantation or explantation. Write down the reasons. Talk with others who have had the same procedure (they are truly the experts!). Look at your expectations: are they realistic? Having implants, or removing implants, may not be a magic solution for you; it may only be part of the solution. [For some more points to consider, see page 206.]

2.   Ask yourself, "Am I educated on the possible side effects of implants?" Evaluating the possible health risks involved is of paramount importance. But women who have had implants also report certain psychological "side effects," such as embarrassment over telling lovers about their implants, handling comments from insensitive friends and family, and a change in physical appearance that can be followed by identity confusion. As we all know, our culture maintains such an identification with our bodies, and for women, this includes an overidentification with the size and appearance of our breasts. We often form a personal sense of self around our breasts, and then when our bodies are altered, we have to be prepared to alter our self-image.

   Look inside yourself to see what fears, concerns, and expectations you have. Run possible scenarios on your own "inner screen" to see how you would feel in certain situations, and if you could comfortably handle those situations. Talk to friends. If need be, talk to a counselor familiar with the issues common to women who have had implants. Be active toward these issues—not just reactive. Seek out experts, read, and contact support groups. These are good measures of self-care and self-respect.

3.   You will look different after implantation/explantation than you do now. How you will look different is an idea in your head that may or may not be matched by the surgery. Can you deal with the unexpected results, positive or negative? For most women having reconstruction, nipples must be constructed from other parts of their bodies. Other women choose not to have this done, and remain nippleless on their reconstructed breast. This requires making a healthy psychological adaptation to the difference between your two breasts, because you will live with this difference every day.

Have you thought about scarring? Often the scars are slight with implantation and more pronounced and extensive with explantation. Here again, every woman is different and should consider her body history and be clear with her doctors about incision size and placement. Explore these visual aspects of the procedures with your intimate others. Viewing pictures will make it more real to both you and your partner(s).

4.   Implantation—and explantation—is major surgery. Do you have the stamina, finances, and support to see yourself through this process? You will need to have all these aspects in place well before the surgery so your energy and focus are on your healing, not on problem solving. *Teach* your friends and family how to support you during this process. Ask for what you need. You will feel vulnerable after the surgery, so don't set yourself up for disappointment and neglect. (I know of one woman having explantation who asked her women friends to give her a shower honoring the "birth" of her smaller breasts. Her friends gifted her with bras, tank tops, and an application for a wet-T-shirt contest. Humor has been proven to be a valuable aid in healing!)

5. Choose your physician carefully. Ask him or her how many of these procedures he or she has actually done. Ask to speak with some of his or her patients who have had similar surgeries. Ask your physician for a step-by-step description of what to expect during pre-op, the operation, and post-op. For example, discuss the anesthesia used and the possible aftereffects. If you are having implants, discuss the materials used in your implants, the safety of those materials, and the possibility of ruptures. If you are undergoing explantation, discuss the changes in your breast size and shape, changes in breast and nipple sensitivity, and scarring. Also ask the following: How long will you be recuperating? What will the healing process entail? Will you need special bras immediately after the surgery? Will you need help at home after the surgery?

If you have difficulty getting the answers to your questions or personal concerns, this person may not be the physician for you. Shop around. Talk to others who have had the surgery. Be sure to look at before-and-after pictures so that your expectations are realistic.

When you have a sense of what you will probably look like after the surgery, do a visualization: Take fifteen minutes, find a quiet place, and make sure you are not disturbed. Sit comfortably, take some deep breaths to relax your body, let go of all thoughts, and simply concentrate on your breathing for a few minutes. Next, imagine yourself, with your new breast(s), standing naked in front of a mirror. Look at yourself from all angles. Look at yourself in different kinds of clothing. Put on a T-shirt...a sweater...a nightgown...a dress. Now "feel" yourself with your new breast(s). Touch them. How do they feel? Are you comfortable with this sense of yourself? Next, look at your whole body. Do you see a balance and a sense of unity to your new physique? Focus your attention on your eyes. Appreciate yourself for the beautiful woman you are. Now gently open your eyes and come back into the room.

Again, it may be helpful to talk with a counselor if you feel an uncomfortable discrepancy between the new image and your current body or if you have conflicts you are struggling to resolve. Knowledge reduces anxiety—and knowledge plus preparation is the best possible foundation for surgery.

*Sharyn Higdon Jones is a licensed marriage and family therapist who practices in San Jose, California. She specializes in sexual abuse, chronic illness, women's issues, and couples counseling. She is a seminar leader and founder of the Healing Steps Workshop Series for sexually abused women. She embraces an eclectic/Jungian approach to inner issues and fosters emotional and spiritual growth in her clients.*

## MORE POINTS TO CONSIDER

Diana Zuckerman, Ph.D., recommends you also take these points into consideration:

◆ When you talk to women who had the procedure, pick women who had it at least 10 years earlier, preferably longer. They are harder to find, but will provide more useful information. And of course, the more women the better.

◆ If you must buy your augmentation on the installment plan (and there are even websites that advertise plans), you can't afford it, because you could have a problem that needs fixing before you've even paid off the surgery. Many women who need explantation can't afford it.

◆ Bear in mind that many plastic surgeons use augmentation photos of women who are not their patients. This common practice was admitted even by a pro-implant plastic surgeon on the FDA advisory panel. (See the FDA transcript, which is linked to the website www.breast-implantinfo.org.)

◆ If you use guided imagery, imagine how you will feel if you get a common complication, such as if your implants get hard or asymmetrical or lose sensation. What will that seem like in intimate encounters?

# Breast-Implant Facts and Figures

## Numbers of Procedures Performed in the United States

Figures for procedures include but are not limited to those performed by members of the American Society of Plastic Surgeons.

| Procedure | 2000 | 1999 | 1997 | Percent Change 1999–2000 | Percent Change 1997–2000 |
|---|---|---|---|---|---|
| Breast augmentation | 203,310 | 191,583 | 101,176 | +6% | +101% |
| Breast lift | 45,710 | 44,861 | 19,882 | +2% | +130% |
| Breast reduction | 90,042 | 89,769 | 47,874 | +0% | +88% |
| Breast reconstruction | 114,497 | 101,228 | 50,337 | +13.1% | +113% |

## Average Fees for the Year 2000

Breast augmentation $4,556
Breast lift $4,658
Breast reduction $5,430
Breast reconstruction $5,430

# References

## Introduction

Kessler, D., R. Merkatz, and R. Shapiro, "A Call for Higher Standards for Breast Implants," *Journal of the American Medical Association*, 1993; 270: 2607–08.

## Chapter 1

Angell, M., "Breast Implants: Protectionism or Paternalism?" *The New England Journal of Medicine*, 18 June 1992; 326(25): 1695–96.

Blakeslee, S., "Implant Maker Had Conflicting Findings on Silicone's Effects," *The New York Times*, 9 May 1994.

Brimelow, P., and L. Spenser, "The Plaintiff Attorneys' Great Honey Rush," *Forbes*, 16 October 1989.

Brimelow, P., and L. Spencer, "Ralph Nader, Inc.," *Forbes*, 17 September 1990.

Hatcher, C., et al., "Breast Cancer and Silicone Implants: Psychological Consequences for Women," *Journal of the National Cancer Institute*, 1 September 1993; 85(17): 1361–65.

Kessler, D., "The Basis of FDA's Decision on Breast Implants," *The New England Journal of Medicine*, 18 June 1992; 326(25): 1713–15.

Regush, N., "Toxic Breasts," *Mother Jones*, January/February 1992, 25–31.

## Chapter 2

Handel, N., et al., "Knowledge, Concern and Satisfaction among Augmentation Mammaplasty Patients," *Annals of Plastic Surgery*, 1993; 30: 13–22.

Leigh, S., and N. Webb, "To Reconstruct or Not to Reconstruct: That Is the Question!" *Innovations in Oncology Nursing*, 1994; 10(1): 1.

Rowland, J., et al., "Type of Breast Cancer Surgery Has Little Impact on Quality of Life," *Journal of the National Cancer Institute*, September 6, 2000; (92)17: 1365.

Winer, E. P., et al., "Silicone Controversy: A Survey of Women with Breast Cancer and Silicone Implants," *Journal of the National Cancer Institute*, 1 September 1993; 85(17): 1407–1411.

## Chapter 3

Anton, M., L. Eskenazi, and C. R. Hartrampf, "Nipple Reconstruction with Local Flaps: Star and Wrap Flaps," *Plastic Surgery*, 1991; 5(1): 67–78.

Bostwick, J., "Breast Reconstruction after Mastectomy: Recent Advances," *Cancer*, 1990; 6: 1402–11.

Clough, K. B., et al., "Prospective Evaluation of Late Cosmetic Results Following Breast Reconstruction," *Plastic and Reconstructive Surgery*, 2001; 107(7): 1702–9.

Elliot, L. F., P. H. Beegle, C. R. Hartrampf, et al., "Breast Reconstruction Following Mastectomy: An Update," *Journal of the Medical Association of Georgia*, 1991; 80: 607–15.

Elliot, L. F., L. Eskenazi, et al., "Immediate TRAM Flap Breast Reconstruction: 128 Consecutive Cases," *Plastic and Reconstructive Surgery*, 1993; 99(2): 217–27.

Ellis, C., "Breast Reconstruction After Mastectomy," *Innovations in Oncology Nursing*, 1994; 10(1): 2–8.

Eskenazi, L., "A One-Stage Nipple Reconstruction with the 'Modified Star' Flap and Immediate Tattoo: A Review of 100 Cases," *Plastic and Reconstructive Surgery*, September 1993; 92(4): 671–80.

Fraulin, F., et al., "Functional Evaluation of the Shoulder Following Latissimus Dorsi Muscle Transfer," presented at the 63rd Annual Meeting of ASPRS, 24–28 September 1994, in *Plastic Surgical Forum*, 17: 228–29.

Hartrampf, C. R., and G. R. Bennett, "Autogenous Tissue Reconstruction in the Mastectomy Patient: A Critical Review of 300 Patients," *Annals of Surgery*, 1987; 205: 508.

Knowlton, E., "The 'Peg' Latissimus Dorsi Flap Procedure: A One-Step Breast Reconstruction," presented at the 63rd Annual Meeting of ASPRS, 24–28 September 1994, in *Plastic Surgical Forum*, 17: 180–81.

Kroll, S. S., "Breast Reconstruction after Mastectomy," *Cancer Bulletin*, 1990; 42: 34–38.

Kroll, S. S., and B. Baldwin, "A Comparison of Outcomes Using Three Different Methods of Breast Reconstruction," *Plastic and Reconstructive Surgery*, September 1992; 90(3): 455–62.

Kroll, S. S., et al., "The Oncologic Risks of Skin Preservation at Mastectomy when Combined with Immediate Reconstruction of the Breast," *Surgery, Gynecology and Obstetrics,* 1991; 172: 17.

Phillips, L., "Reconstructive Options Following Mastectomy," *Journal of the American Medical Women's Association,* September/October 1992; 47(5): 178–80.

Rosen, P. B., et al., "Clinical Experience with Immediate Breast Reconstruction Using Tissue Expansion or Transverse Rectus Abdominis Musculotaneous Flaps," *Annals of Plastic Surgery,* 1990; 25: 249.

Shaw, W. W., "Breast Reconstruction by Superior Gluteal Microvascular Free Flaps Without Silicone Implants," *Plastic and Reconstructive Surgery,* 1983; 72: 490.

## Chapter 4

Birdsell, D. C., et al., "Breast Cancer Diagnosis and Survival in Women with and Without Breast Implants," *Plastic and Reconstructive Surgery,* October 1993; 92(5): 795–800.

Brown, L., et al., "Prevalence of Rupture of Silicone-Gel Breast Implants Revealed on MR Imaging in a Population of Women in Birmingham, Alabama," *American Journal of Roentgenology,* 2000; 175: 1057–64.

Burton, T. M., "Doctors See Hazards in Breast Implants Despite What Recent Studies May Say," *The Wall Street Journal,* 24 August 1994.

"Debate over Breast Implants and Imaging," *ACR Bulletin,* May 1989; 34: 10.

Dershaw, D. D., and T. A. Chaglassian, "Mammography after Prosthesis Placement for Augmentation or Reconstruction Mammaplasty," *Radiology,* 1989; 170: 69–74.

Eklund, G. W., et al., "Improved Imaging of the Augmented Breast," *American Journal of Radiology,* 1988; 151: 469–73.

"FDA Proposes Mandatory Informed Consent Prior to Breast Implants," *ACR Bulletin,* February 1989; 45: 8.

Fisher, J. C., "The Silicone Controversy: When Will Science Prevail?" *The New England Journal of Medicine,* 18 June 1992; 326(25): 1696–98.

Handel, N., M. Silverstein, and P. Gamagami, "The Effect of Breast Implants on Mammography and Cancer Detection," *Perspectives in Plastic Surgery,* 1993; 7(1): 1–31.

Pagnozzi, A., "Why Does the Media Let Women Believe Breast Implants Are Safe?" *Glamour,* September 1994, 172.

Reintgen, D., et al., "The Anatomy of Missed Breast Cancers," *Surgical Oncology*, 1993; 2: 65–75.

Silverstein, M. J., N. Handel, P. Gamagami, et al., "Breast Cancer Diagnosis and Prognosis in Women Following Augmentation with Silicone-Gel-Filled Prostheses," *European Journal of Cancer*, 1992; 28: 635.

Wolfe, S., "Implant Study Too Small for Final Word," letter to *The New York Times*, 28 June 1994.

Young, V. L., et al., "Biocompatibility of Radiolucent Breast Implants," *Plastic and Reconstructive Surgery*, September 1991; 88(3): 462–74.

Young, V. L., et al., "Effect of Breast Implants on Mammography," *Southern Medical Journal*, June 1991; 84(6): 707–14.

## Chapter 5

Berkel, H., et al., "Breast Augmentation: A Risk Factor for Breast Cancer?" *The New England Journal of Medicine*, 1992; 326(25): 1649–53.

Blakeslee, S., "An Anti-Cancer Role Is Hinted for Silicone," *The New York Times*, 10 August 1994.

Borenstein, D., "Siliconosis: A Spectrum of Illness," *Seminars in Arthritis and Rheumatism*, August 1994; 24(1), Supplement 1: 1–7.

Brautbar, N., "Silicone Breast Implants and Autoimmunity: Causation or Myth?" *Archives of Environmental Health*, May/June 1994; 49(3): 151–53.

Brautbar, N., et al., "Silicone Implants and Systemic Immunological Disease: Review of the Literature and Preliminary Results," *Toxicology and Industrial Health*, 1992; 8(5): 231–37.

Bridges, A. J., et al., "A Clinical and Immunologic Evaluation of Women with Silicone Breast Implants and Symptoms of Rheumatic Disease," *Annals of Internal Medicine*, 1993; 118(12): 929–36.

Brinton, L., et al., "Breast Cancer Following Augmentation Mammoplasty," *Cancer Causes and Control*, 2000; 11(9): 819–27.

Brinton, L., et al., "Cancer Risk at Sites Other than the Breast Following Augmentation Mammoplasty," *Annals of Epidemiology*, 2001; 11: 248–56.

Burton, T., "Breast Implants Raise More Safety Issues," *The Wall Street Journal*, 4 February 1993.

Deapan, D., and G. Brody, "Augmentation Mammoplasty and Breast Cancer: A Five-Year Update of the Los Angeles Study," *Plastic and Reconstructive Surgery*, April 1992; 89(4): 660–65.

Deapan, D., et al., "Are Breast Implants Anticarcinogenic? A Fourteen-Year Follow-Up of the Los Angeles Study," *Plastic and Reconstructive Surgery,* 1997; 99: 1346–53.

Deapan, D., et al., "Breast Cancer Stage at Diagnosis and Survival among Patients with Prior Breast Implants," *Plastic and Reconstructive Surgery,* 2000; 105: 535–40.

Dowden, R., "Periprosthetic Bacteria and the Breast Implant Patient with Systemic Symptoms," *Plastic and Reconstructive Surgery,* August 1994; 94(2): 300–5.

Epstein, S., "Women at Risk Are Still in the Dark," *Los Angeles Times,* 9 September 1994.

Fisher, J. C., "The Silicone Controversy: When Will Science Prevail?" *The New England Journal of Medicine,* 18 June 1992; 326(25): 1696–98.

Freundlich, B., et al., "A Profile of Symptomatic Patients with Silicone Breast Implants: A Sjögrens-Like Syndrome," *Seminars in Arthritis and Rheumatism,* August 1994; 24(91), Supplement: 44–53.

Friemann, J., et al., "Physiologic and pathologic patterns of reactions to silicone breast implants," *Zentralbl Chir,* 1997; 122:7, 551–564.

Frost, E., "Breast Implant Cancer Link Alleged," *American Bar Association Journal,* June 1991; 18.

Gabriel, S., et al., "Risk of Connective-Tissue Diseases and Other Disorders after Breast Implantation," *New England Journal of Medicine,* 16 June 1994; 330(24): 1697–1702.

Goldblum, R. M., R. P. Pelley, et al., "Antibodies to Silicone Elastomers and Reactions to Ventriculoperitoneal Shunts," *Lancet,* 1992; 340: 510.

Hilts, Philip, "New Risk Is Found in Breast Implants," *The New York Times,* 25 September 1993.

Hilts, Philip, "Two Studies Link Breast Implants and Antibodies," *The New York Times,* 20 March 1993.

Kasper, C. S., "Histologic features of breast capsules reflect surface configuration and composition of silicone bag implants," *American Journal of Clinical Pathology,* November 1994; 102:5, 655–659.

Kolata, G., "Scleroderma and Breast Devices: No Tie Seen," *The New York Times,* 29 May 1994.

Kolata, G., "Study Finds Nothing to Link Implants with Any Diseases," *The New York Times,* 16 June 1994.

Kossovsky, N., and J. Stassi, "A Pathophysiological Examination of the

Biophysics and Bioreactivity of Silicone Breast Implants," *Seminars in Arthritis and Rheumatism,* August 1994; 24(1), Supplement 1: 18–21.

Ostermeyer Shoaib, B., B. M. Patten, and D. S. Calkins, "Adjuvant Breast Disease: An Evaluation of 100 Symptomatic Women with Breast Implants or Silicone Fluid Injections," *Keio Journal of Medicine,* June 1994; 43(2): 79–87.

Peters, W., et al., "Analysis of silicone levels in capsules of gel and saline implants and penile prostheses," *Annals of Plastic Surgery,* June 1995; 34:6, 578–584.

Press, R., et al., "Antinuclear Autoantibodies in Women with Silicone Breast Implants," *Lancet,* 1992; 340: 1204–7.

Salmon, S. E., and R. A. Kyle, "Silicone Gels, Induction of Plasma Cell Tumors, and Genetic Susceptibility in Mice: A Call for Epidemiological Investigation of Women with Silicone Breast Implants," *Journal of the National Cancer Institute,* July 1994; 86: 14.

Schnur, P. L., et al., "Silicone Analysis of Breast and Periprosthetic Capsular Tissue from Patients with Saline or Silicone-Gel Breast Implants," presented at the 63rd Annual Meeting of ASPRS, 24–28 September 1994, in *Plastic Surgical Forum,* 17: 200–2.

Silverstein, M. J., N. Handel, and P. Gamagami, et al., "Breast Cancer Diagnosis and Prognosis in Women Following Augmentation with Silicone-Gel-Filled Prostheses," *European Journal of Cancer,* 1992; 28: 635.

Smalley, D., et al., "Immunologic Stimulation of Lymphocytes in Silicone Breast Implant Patients," "Immunologic Stimulation of Lymphocytes in Silicone-Gel Breast-Implant Patients and Their Children," "Anamnestic Immune Response to Silica Following Re-exposure in a Mammary Implant Patient," and other unpublished papers; call (800) 280-1278 for abstracts.

Solomon, G., "A Clinical and Laboratory Profile of Symptomatic Women with Silicone Breast Implants," *Seminars in Arthritis and Rheumatism,* August 1994; 24(1), Supplement: 29–37.

Spiera, H., "Scleroderma after Silicone Augmentation Mammaplasty," *Journal of the American Medical Association,* 1988; 260: 236–8.

Spiera, H., and L. D. Kerr, "Scleroderma Following Silicone Implantation: A Cumulative Experience of Eleven Cases," *The Journal of Rheumatology,* 1993; 20(6): 958–61.

Spiera, R. F., A. Gibofsky, and H. Spiera, "Silicone-Gel-Filled Breast Implants and Connective-Tissue Disease: An Overview," *The Journal of Rheumatology,* 1994; 21: 239–45.

Swan, S. H., "Epidemiology of Silicone-Related Disease," *Seminars in Arthritis and Rheumatism*, August 1994; 24(1), Supplement 1: 38–43.

Teuber S. S., R. L. Saunders, G. M. Halpern, R. F. Brucker, V. Conte, B. D. Goldman, E. E. Winger, W. G. Wood, and M. E. Gershwin. "Serum silicon levels are elevated in women with silicone gel implants." *Current Topics in Microbiology and Immunology*. 1996; 210: 59–65.

Vasey, F. B., et al., "Clinical Findings in Symptomatic Women with Silicone Breast Implants," *Seminars in Arthritis and Rheumatism*, August 1994; (24)1, Supplement 1: 22–28.

Vojdani, A., N. Brautbar, and A. W. Campbell, "Antibody to Silicone and Native Macromolecules in Women with Silicone Breast Implants," *Immunopharmacology and Immunotoxicology*, 1994; (16)4 (in press).

Vojdani, A., A. Campbell, and N. Brautbar, "Immune Functional Impairment in Patients with Clinical Abnormalities and Silicone Breast Implants," *Toxicology and Industrial Health*, 1992; (8)6: 415–28.

Yoshida S. H., C. C. Chang, S. S. Teuber, M. E. Gershwin. "Silicon and silicone: theoretical and clinical implications of breast implants." *Regulatory Toxicology and Pharmacology*. 1993 Feb; 17(1): 3–18. Review.

Yoshida S. H., S. S. Teuber, J. B. German, M. E. Gershwin. "Immunotoxicity of silicone: implications of oxidant balance towards adjuvant activity." *Food and Chemical Toxicology*. 1994 Nov; 32(11): 1089–100. Review.

Yoshida S. H., S. Swan, S. S. Teuber, M. E. Gershwin. "Silicone breast implants: immunotoxic and epidemiologic issues." *Life Sciences*. 1995 Mar 10; 56(16): 1299–310. Review.

## Chapter 6

Blakeslee, S., "Blood Tests for Leaks from Implants Raise Questions and Hopes," *The New York Times*, 28 December 1993.

Blais, P. "Residual capsule and intercapsular debris as long-term risk factors." Available at http://explantation.com.

Brucker, R. F., et al., "Elevated Blood Serum Silicon Levels in Women with Silicone-Gel Breast Implants Suspected of Leakage," unpublished; available from Balco Laboratories, (800) 777-7122.

Dobke, M. K., and M. S. Middleton, "Clinical Impact of Breast-Implant Magnetic Resonance Imaging," *Annals of Plastic Surgery*, 1994; 33: 241–46.

Eklund, G. W., et al., "Improved Imaging of the Augmented Breast," *American Journal of Radiology*, 1988; 151: 469–73.

"Fire and Fury," CNN, newsmagazine show about dubious silicone-disease treatments. Aired on 16 October 1994.

Frondoff, S., "Silicone Implants and the Global Settlement," *Breast Cancer Action Newsletter,* April 1994; no. 23, 1.

Gard, Z. R., and E. Brown, "Silicone Breast Implants and Immunological Disease," *Townsend Letter for Doctors,* June 1993; 570–73.

Handel, N., M. Silverstein, and P. Gamagami, "The Effect of Breast Implants on Mammography and Cancer Detection," *Perspectives in Plastic Surgery,* 1993; 7(1): 1–31.

Hardt, N. S., et al., "Complications related to retained breast implant capsules," *Plastic and Reconstructive Surgery Journal,* February 1995; 95: 2: 364–371.

Kossovsky, N., and J. Stassi, "A Pathophysiological Examination of the Biophysics and Bioreactivity of Silicone Breast Implants," *Seminars in Arthritis and Rheumatism,* August 1994; 24(1), Supplement 1: 18–21.

Kron, J., "Breasts to Go," *Allure,* October 1994; 92–98.

Levine, J. J., and N. Ilowite, "Sclerodermalike Esophageal Disease in Children Breast-Fed by Mothers with Silicone Breast Implants," *Journal of the American Medical Association,* 1994; 271: 213–216. See also letters to the editor in 272: 767–770.

Middleton, M. S., "Magnetic Resonance Evaluation of Breast Implants and Soft-Tissue Silicone," *Topics in Magnetic Resonance Imaging,* 1998; 9(2): 92–137.

Rockwell, W. Bradford, et al., "Breast Capsule Persistence after Breast Implant Removal," *Plastic and Reconstructive Surgery Journal,* 1998; 101: 1085.

Rosculet, K., "Ruptured Gel-Filled Silicone Breast Implants: Sonographic Findings in Nineteen Cases," *American Journal of Radiology,* October 1992; 159: 711–716.

Shanklin, D. R., "Letter to insurance company regarding necessity of a total capsulectomy," September 1996. Available at http://explantation.com.

Teuber S. S., R. L. Saunders, G. M. Halpern, R. F. Brucker, V. Conte, B. D. Goldman, E. E. Winger, W. G. Wood, and M. E. Gershwin. "Serum silicon levels are elevated in women with silicone gel implants." *Current Topics in Microbiology and Immunology.* 1996; 210: 59–65.

Vojdani, A., et al., "Immunologic and Biologic Markers for Silicone," *Toxicology and Industrial Health,* 1994; 10(1/2): 25–42.

Vojdani, A., et al., "Laboratory Tests in Aid for Diagnosis of Silicone-

Induced Immunological Disorders: A Review," *Journal of Occupational Medicine and Toxicology,* 1994; 3(1): 1–19.

## Chapter 7

Elias, M., "Transferring Fat to Breasts Poses Risk," *USA Today,* 6 October 1992.

Rosenthal, E., "Female Image of the Male Ideal, in a Faulty Mirror," *The New York Times,* 22 July 1992.

Tong, W. T., "Breast Augmentation by Acupuncture" (letter), *The Medical Journal of Australia,* 10 January 1981.

## Chapter 8

Handel, N., M. Silverstein, and P. Gamagami, "The Effect of Breast Implants on Mammography and Cancer Detection," *Perspectives in Plastic Surgery,* 1993; 7(1): 1–31.

Harcourt, D., and N. Rumsey, "Psychological aspects of breast reconstruction: a review of the literature," *Journal of Advances in Nursing,* August 2001; 35(4): 477–487.

Leigh, S., and N. Webb, "To Reconstruct or Not to Reconstruct: That Is the Question!" *Innovations in Oncology Nursing,* 1994; 10(1): 1.

## Chapter 9

Angell, M., "Breast Implants: Protectionism or Paternalism?" *The New England Journal of Medicine,* 18 June 1992; 326(25): 1695–96.

Blakeslee, S., "Implant Maker Had Conflicting Findings on Silicone's Effects," *The New York Times,* 9 May 1994.

Friedman, R. M., et al., "Saline Made Viscous with PEG: A New Breast Prosthesis," presented at the 63rd Annual Meeting of ASPRS, 24–28 September 1994, in *Plastic Surgical Forum,* 17: 198.

Ketch, L., et al., "HLA Typing and Silicone-Associated Autoimmunity," presented at the 63rd Annual Meeting of ASPRS, 24–28 September 1994, in *Plastic Surgical Forum,* 17: 196.

Kron, J., "Breasts to Go," *Allure,* October 1994; 92–98.

Young, V. Leroy, et al., "Biocompatibility of Radiolucent Breast Implants," *Plastic and Reconstructive Surgery,* September 1991; 88(3): 462–474.

# Bibliography

## Books

The FDA's Regulation of Silicone Breast Implants, December 1992. Staff report by the Human Resources and Intergovernmental Relations Subcommittee of the Committee on Government Operations. U.S. Government Printing Office, 1993.

Guthrie, Randolph H., with Doug Podolsky. *The Truth about Breast Implants.* New York: John Wiley and Sons, 1994.

Jenny, Henry. *Silicone-Gate: Exposing the Breast Implant Scandal.* Siloam Springs, 1994. (To order, call (800) 574-2978.)

Lappe, Mark. *Chemical Deception: The Toxic Threat to Health and the Environment.* San Francisco: Sierra Club Books, 1991. See especially the chapter on nonreactive chemicals.

Lorant, Terry, photographer, with text by Loren Eskenazi. *Reconstructing Aphrodite.* Burlington, VT: Verve Editions, 2001. (To order, call (802) 860-2866.)

Love, Susan M. *Dr. Susan Love's Breast Book.* Reading, MA: Addison-Wesley Publishing Co., 2000 (revised).

Morgan, Elizabeth. *The Complete Book of Cosmetic Surgery.* New York: Warner Books, 1988.

Moynahan, Paula A. *Dr. Paula Moynahan's Cosmetic Surgery for Women.* New York: Crown Publishers, 1988.

Oldt, Linda. *Mad Money: How to Preserve, Protect, and Multiply Your Personal-Injury Lawsuit Settlement.* Winter Haven, FL: Investment Information Associates. (To order, call (800) 785-5228.)

Rosenthal, Ilena. *Breast Implants: The Myths, The Facts, The Women.* Self-published; available from: Ilena Rosenthal, 1380 Garnet #444, San Diego, CA 92109 (please include a $20 donation).

Rothfleisch, Sheldon. *The No-Nonsense Guide to Cosmetic Surgery.* New York: Grosset and Dunlap, 1979.

Snyder, Marilyn. *An Informed Decision: Understanding Breast Reconstruction.* New York: M. Evans, 1989.

Vasey, Frank, and Josh Feldstein. *The Silicone Breast Implant Controversy.* Freedom, CA: The Crossing Press, 1993.

Wolfe, Sidney. *Women's Health Alert.* Reading, MA: Addison-Wesley Publishing Co., 1991. Coauthored by the Public Citizen Health Research Group; includes a chapter on breast implants called "Time Bombs Ticking."

## Miscellaneous

"Are Breast Implants Safe?" by Diana Zuckerman. Medscape General Medicine. <http://www.medscape.com/viewarticle/408187>. 2001; 3(4).

"The Breast Cancer Information Gap," by Diana Zuckerman. *RN Magazine.* 2002; 65(2): 39-41.

"The Breast Implant Controversy," by Ralph R. Cook, et al. *Arthritis and Rheumatism.* February 1994; 37(2): 153–57.

"Breast Implants: What Price Vanity?" by Doug Podolsky. *American Health.* March 1991; 70–75.

"Breast Implant Special Report," The National Women's Health Resource Center. March/April 1992; 14(2): 1-9.

"Controversy over the Silicone-Gel Breast Implant: Current Status and Clinical Implications," by Rod Rohrich and Clifford Clark. *Texas Medicine: The Journal.* September 1993; 89(9): 53–58.

"Facts about Implants and Their Safety," editorial by Jean Paul Bosse, M.D. *International Confederation of Plastic and Reconstructive Surgeons Newsletter.* April 1992.

"Image of Perfection Once the Goal—Now Some Women Just Seek Damages." *Journal of the American Medical Association.* 13 May 1992; 2439–2442.

"Is There a Time Bomb Ticking in Women's Breasts?" by Carla Rohlfing. *Longevity.* July 1991; 52–58.

"The Political and Social Context of Silicone Breast Implant Use in the United States," by Jane Sprague Zones. *Journal of Long-Term Effects of Medical Implants.* 1992; 1(3): 225–241.

"Postmastectomy Breast Reconstruction: Recent Advances and Controversies," by Cynthia Booth Lord. *Clinician Reviews.* November/December 1991; 43–69.

"Replacing the Irreplaceable," by Sue Mittenthal. *New York*. November 12, 1984, 94-111.

❖ ❖ ❖

Food and Drug Administration: various documents relating to implants.

Information packets from: Command Trust Network, Public Citizen Health Research Group, National Women's Health Network.

Patient education brochures from McGhan and Mentor.

Various articles in *The Washington Post, The New York Times,* and *The Wall Street Journal.*

# Resources

Here is contact information for the major groups and institutions involved in breast-implant regulation, surgery, and information. You can get an amazing amount of information via the Internet, as well as find online support groups, chat rooms, and bulletin boards. Of course, the telephone and conventional mail still work, too.

## Food and Drug Administration

The FDA's Office of Health and Industry Programs (OHIP) is responsible for answering breast-implant calls and distributing the official breast-implant handbook. To receive a copy of the breast-implant handbook, contact their Consumer Affairs Staff at (888) 463-6332.

You may also obtain the breast-implant handbook by visiting the FDA's website at: www.fda.gov/cdrh/breastimplants/indexbip.html.

For additional information, visit another FDA website at: www.fda.gov/cdrh/consumer/index.html. Click on "Products Regulated," then click on the letter B, and scroll down to "Breast Implants."

You may also wish to contact the following for more information:

**Food and Drug Administration**
Office of Consumer Affairs
5600 Fishers Ln., Rm. 16-59
Rockville MD 20857        (888) INFO-FDA

**Food and Drug Administration**
Office of Women's Health
5600 Fishers Ln., Rm. 14-62
Rockville MD 20857

**MEDWATCH**              (800) FDA-1088 (382-1088)
Call for adverse-reaction forms.

## Other Federal-Government Resources

**Medicare Hotline**         (800) MEDICARE

**Institute of Medicine Report**

The Institute of Medicine (IOM) report, Safety of Silicone Breast Implants, is available for sale from:

National Academy Press
2101 Constitution Ave. NW,
Box 285
Washington DC 20055    (800) 624-6242 or (202) 334-3938

You may also purchase the report through the Internet at http://books. nap.edu/catalog/9602.html or read it at the same website for free.

A consumer booklet on the IOM study, Information for Women about the Safety of Silicone Breast Implants, can be purchased from the National Academy of Sciences on their website at: http://books.nap.edu/ catalog/9618.html or read it at the same website for free.

These reports do not include the 2001 studies from the FDA and NCI, or the local complication data from the FDA meeting in 2000. These and other studies are available on the Internet at www. breastimplantinfo.org; www.toxic-exposure.com; and www.toxicdiscov ery.com/informed_consent.htm.

## *Women's Health*

**National Association for Women's Health**
300 N. Adams, Ste. 328
Chicago IL 60606-5101    (312) 786-1468
Fax: (312) 786-0376    E-mail: fbloom@nawh.org

**National Women's Health Network**
514 Tenth St. NW, Ste. 400
Washington DC 20004
(202) 347-1140    Fax: (202) 347-1168
Website: www.womenshealthnetwork.org

For a small fee, they will send you information packets on saline and silicone breast implants (as well an array of other health topics) containing a glossary, resource list, an average of three to five articles, and extensive annotated bibliographies.

**National Women's Health Resource Center**
120 Albany St., Ste. 820
New Brunswick NJ 08901    (877) 986-9472
Fax: (732) 249-4671    Website: www.healthywomen.org

**National Center for Policy Research (CPR) for Women & Families**
1901 Pennsylvania Ave., NW, Ste. 901
Washington DC 20006    (202) 223-4000
website: www.center4policy.org

**Public Citizen Health Research Group**
1600 20th St. NW
Washington DC 20009          (202) 588-1000
Website: www.citizen.org

**Boston Women's Health Book Collective**
PO Box 192
West Somerville MA 02144
617) 625-0277               Fax: (617) 625-0294

## *Plastic, Cosmetic, and Reconstructive Surgeons*

**American Society of Plastic Surgeons (ASPS; formerly ASPRS)**
444 East Algonquin Rd.
Arlington Heights IL 60005     (888) 4-PLASTIC (475-2784)
Website: www.plasticsurgery.org

**American Society for Aesthetic Plastic Surgery**
11081 Winners Circle, Ste. 200
Los Alamitos CA 90710       (888) 272-7711
Fax: (562) 799-1098         Website: www.surgery.org/home.asp

**American Academy of Cosmetic Surgery**
401 N. Michigan Ave.
Chicago IL 60611-4267       (312) 527-6713
Fax: (312) 644-1815         E-mail: aacs@spa.com
Website: www.cosmeticsurgery.org

**American College of Surgeons**
633 N. St. Claire St.
Chicago IL 60611            (312) 202-5000
Fax: (312) 202-5001         Website: www.facs.org

**American Society of Plastic and Reconstructive Surgical Nurses**
East Holly Ave., Box 56
Pitman NJ 08071-0056        (609) 256-2340
Fax: (609) 489-7463         Website: http://asprsn.inurse.com

## *Breast Cancer, and Cancer Generally*

**National Cancer Institute**
Office of Cancer Communications, Bldg. 31, Rm. 10A-24
9000 Rockville Pike
Bethesda MD 20892           (800) 4-CANCER (422-6237)

**Y-ME National Breast Cancer Organization**
212 W. Van Buren

Chicago IL 60607-3908      (800) 221-2141
Fax: (312) 294-8597      Website: www.y-me.org
This breast cancer information and support service provides telephone counseling and answers to questions about breast cancer and reconstruction; customized consumer- and patient-oriented information packets are available by mail.

**Hope Line**      (703) 461-9616
This affiliate of Y-ME, located in the greater Washington, D.C., area, matches and connects women with others who've had similar breast cancer experiences for support and information sharing.

**Cancer Information Service**    (800) 4-CANCER (422-6237)
A service of the National Cancer Institute. Trained nonphysician cancer-information specialists answer questions about breast cancer treatment; services in English and Spanish.

**American Cancer Society**
1599 Clifton Rd. NE
Atlanta GA 30329      (800) ACS-2345
(or check telephone directory for your local chapter)
Website: www.cancer.org
Offers counseling and information about options after mastectomy; referral available to local sources for prostheses and plastic surgeons.

**Breast Cancer Action**
55 New Montgomery, Ste. 323
San Francisco CA 94105      (415) 243-9301

**National Breast Cancer Coalition**
1707 L St. NW, Ste. 1060
Washington DC 20036      (202) 296-7477

**National Alliance of Breast Cancer Organizations**
9 East 37th St., 10th Fl.
New York NY 10016      (212) 889-0606
Fax: (212) 939-1213      E-mail: Nabco.info@aol.com
Website: www.nabco.org

**Cancer Hope Network**
Two North Rd.
Chester NJ 07930      (877) HOPENET (467-3638)
E-mail: info@cancerhopenetwork.org
Provides free, confidential, one-on-one support to people with cancer and their families. Matches patients with trained volunteers who have themselves undergone a similar experience. Provides support and hope

to help patients and families look beyond the diagnosis, cope with treatment, and start living life to its fullest once again.

**The Susan G. Komen Breast Cancer Foundation**
5005 LBJ Freeway, Ste. 250
Dallas TX 75244                     (972) 855-1600
(800) 462-9273 (help line)      Fax: (972) 855-1605
E-mail: Breast health or breast cancer concerns: helpline@komen.org
          Educational programs or materials: education@komen.org

## Breast Self-Exam Reminder

To remind you about monthly breast self-exam, the Susan G. Komen Foundation has available a two-sided, four-color, five-inch-by-ten-inch waterproof card that describes and illustrates the steps of breast self-examination (BSE) in both English and Spanish. It features punch-out BSE reminder dots for each month. The card, designed to hang in your shower, is free and can be obtained by calling the help line (above); or it can be ordered in bulk (250 cards) for $62.50, plus shipping and handling, by calling (877) SGK-SHOP (754-7467).

## Silicone-Implant Organizations: Information, Support, Advocacy

There is a proliferation of silicone groups, newsletters, and meetings. Contact one or more of the following and you will be hooked into the network of women and their families, interested and knowledgeable physicians, and the latest developments on all fronts.

**Implant Information Project**
National Center for Policy Research for Women and Families
1901 Pennsylvania Ave., NW, Suite 901
Washington DC 20006          (202) 223-4000
Website: www.breastimplantinfo.org or www.center4policy.org

**Life After Breast Implants**
Website: http://community-1.webtv.net/lany25/LifeAfterBreast0/
This website offers women's stories, scientific articles about breast implants, and additional breast implant links, including treatment protocols tried by silicone survivors, Dow Corning contact addresses, and other information for the breast implant litigation case.

The web producers have also created Breast Augmentation and Reconstruction, (BAAR) a public newsletter providing information about breast augmentation and reconstruction surgeries, including breast implants and tissue transfer surgery.

Website: http://groups.yahoo.com/group/BreastAugmentationAndRecon-
struction

**Central Texas Silicone-Implant Support, Inc.**
1900A Gracy Farms Ln.
Austin TX 78758          Phone/Fax: (512) 837-5254
E-mail: jcraig@realtime.net

**Coalition of Silicone Survivors (COSS)**
Contact: Lynda Roth
PO Box 129
Broomfield CO 80038-0129     (970) 506-9288
Fax: (970) 506-9288          E-mail: coss1@uswest.net

**Humantics Foundation for Women**
Breast Implants: Recovery and Discovery
Contact: Ilena Rose
1380 Garnet #444
San Diego CA 92109           (858) 270-0680
E-mail: Ilena@san.rr.com or ilena2000@hotmail.com
Website: www.info-implants.com/Quebec/Espoir/03.html
*or* www.toxic-exposure.com

**Implant Information Foundation**
PO Box 2907
Laguna Hills CA 92653

**The Silicone Survivors Support Network**
PO Box 117
Fairhope AL 36532            (334) 928-7731

**National Breast-Implant Task Force**
PO Box 210503
West Palm Beach FL 33414     (561) 791-2625
                             Fax: (561) 791-4419

**Toxic Discovery Network, Inc.**
1906 Grant Ln.
Columbia MO 65203
(573) 445-0861               Fax: (573) 445-0861
E-mail: toxicdiscovery@plateauconsulting.com
*or* breastimplantinfo@plateauconsulting.com
Website: www.plateauconsulting.com/toxicdiscoverynetwork
*or* www.toxicdiscovery.com/informed_consent.htm

**United Silicone Survivors of the World, Houston Chapter**
12615 Misty Valley
Houston TX 77066                     (281) 444-4796
Fax: (281) 444-5468                  E-mail: keeling.m@att.net

**Plaintiffs' Liaison Council**
2008 Second Ave., N.
Birmingham AL 35203                  (205) 252-6784
Fax: (205) 252-0423                  E-mail: dburchfield@breastimplant.org

**Breast Augmentation and Breast Implants Information Website by Nicole**
Website: www.implantinfo.com
This website allows visitors to share positive experiences, opinions, and information on breast implants, breast augmentation, breast enlargement, plastic surgery and recovery.

## Disease-Specific Organizations

**Arthritis Foundation**
PO Box 7669
Atlanta GA 30357-0069                (800) 283-7800
(404) 872-7100, ext. 6350            Website: www.arthritis.org

**National Chronic Fatigue Syndrome and Myalgia Association**
PO Box 18426
Kansas City MO 64133                 (816) 931-4777

**National Multiple Sclerosis Society**
205 E. 42nd St.
New York NY 10028                    (800) 227-3166

**Scleroderma Foundation**
89 Newbury St.
Danvers MA 01923                     (800) 722-HOPE
E-mail: sfinfo@scleroderma.org Fax: (978) 750-9902
Website: www.scleroderma.org

**Fibromyalgia Network**
5700 Stockdale Hwy., Ste. 100
Bakersfield CA 93309

**Lupus Foundation of America**
1300 Piccard Dr., Ste. 200
Rockville MD 20850                   (800) 558-0121
Fax: (301) 670-9486                  E-mail: lupusinfo@aol.com

**CANDO (Chemically Associated/Neurological Disorders)**
PO Box 682633
Houston TX 77268-2633    (281) 444-0662
Fax: (281) 444-5468    E-mail: keeling.m@worldnet.att.net

## Children's Issues

**La Leche League International**
9616 Minneapolis Ave.
PO Box 1209
Franklin Park IL 60131-8209    (708) 455-7730
Information for mothers who breast-feed.

**Children Afflicted by Toxic Substances (CATS)**
413 Fort Salonga Rd.
Northport NY 11768    (631) 757-4829
Fax: (631) 757-4872    E-mail: catstoxic@aol.com

**Toxic 2 KIDS**
915 Rustic Dr.
Macon MO 63552    (660) 385-4621
Fax: (660) 385-3289
On-line Newsgroup: toxic2kids@egroups.com
E-mail: (chair, Cindy Fuchs-Morrissey) Fuchs/Morrissey@hotmail.com
(co-chair, Ed Brent) brentko@mindspring.com
Website: www.plateauconsulting.com/toxicdiscoverynetwork/toxickids.
html

## Treatment Clinics

**American Holistic Medical Association**
Contact: Susan Kolb, M.D., FACS
6728 Old McLean Village Dr.
McLean VA 22101

For an AHMA referral directory, send a check or money order for $10.
Call or e-mail the silicone support groups listed above and ask for recommendations.

## Manufacturers of Implants

**Mentor Corporation**
201 Mentor Dr.
Santa Barbara CA 93111    (800) MENTOR-8 (636-8678)
Website: www.mentorcorp.com

**McGhan**
700 Ward Dr.
Santa Barbara CA 93111　　(800) 624-4261
Website: www.mcghan.com

## Manufacturers of Prostheses

### External Prostheses and "Falsies"

**Cactus Point L.L.C.**
PO Box 3757
Rapid City SD 57709　　Fax: (605) 341-5401
E-mail: info@cpmart.com　　Website: www.cpmart.com
Order from the website, or via e-mail, snail-mail, or fax.

**Nearly You**
Call or fax your order at: (972) 722-6168
Website: www.nearlyou.com

### Custom Prostheses

**Belle-Amie**
17815 Sky Park Circle, Ste. J
Irvine CA 92614　　(800) 700-2807, (949) 756-9512
Fax: (949) 756-1911　　E-mail: belleami@pacbell.net
Website: www.belle-amie.com
Call or e-mail for a free brochure and free private consultation or to speak to a representative; or visit the website.

# Index

**LYMPHEDEMA: A Breast Cancer Patient's Guide to Prevention and Healing** by Jeannie Burt & Gwen White, P.T.

Thirty percent of all breast cancer survivors in the U.S. may get lymphedema after surgery or radiation. This book emphasizes active self-help—more than 50 illustrations explain treatment procedures, bandaging techniques, and exercises to make treatment more effective. Chapters cover garments, pumps, diet, the effects of environmental chemicals, and the benefits of relaxation. Personal stories highlight practical issues and factors in success.

*"Finally, here is a superbly informative and useful book about lymphedema...."*
— National Lymphedema Network Newsletter

*224 pages ... 50 illus. ... Paperback $12.95 ... Hardcover $22.95*

**RECOVERING FROM BREAST SURGERY: Exercises to Strengthen Your Body and Relieve Pain** by Diana Stumm, P.T.

Very few books specifically address how to eliminate the pain and loss of mobility that follows a mastectomy or other breast surgery. Diana Stumm has worked with women recovering from breast surgery for more than 30 years. She discusses the best exercises for mastectomy, lumpectomy, radiation, reconstruction, and lymphedema. Clear drawings illustrate specific stretches, massage techniques, and exercises that form the crucial steps to a full and pain-free recovery.

*"[Diana Stumm's] knowledge of breast cancer management is unsurpassed in the world of physical therapy."*
— Francis A. Marzoni, Jr., M.D.

*128 pages ... 25 illus. ... Paperback ... $11.95*

**THE FEISTY WOMAN'S BREAST CANCER BOOK**
by Elaine Ratner    *Featured in* **The New York Times**

This personal, advice-packed guide helps women navigate the emotional and psychological landscape surrounding breast cancer, and make their own decisions with confidence. Its insight and positive message make this a perfect companion for every feisty woman who wants not only to survive but to thrive after breast cancer.

*"There are times when a woman needs a wise and level-headed friend, someone kind, savvy and caring... [This] book is just such a friend..."* — Rachel Naomi Remen, M.D., author of *Kitchen Table Wisdom*

*288 pages ... Paperback $14.95 ... Hardcover $24.95*

# ORDER FORM

10% DISCOUNT on orders of $50 or more —
20% DISCOUNT on orders of $150 or more —
30% DISCOUNT on orders of $500 or more —
*On cost of books for fully prepaid orders*

NAME

ADDRESS

CITY/STATE                                              ZIP/POSTCODE

PHONE                              COUNTRY (outside of U.S.)

| TITLE | QTY | PRICE | TOTAL |
|---|---|---|---|
| Breast Implants 3rd. edition... (paperback) | | @ $12.95 | |

*Prices subject to change without notice*

Please list other titles below:

| | | | |
|---|---|---|---|
| | | @ $ | |
| | | @ $ | |
| | | @ $ | |
| | | @ $ | |
| | | @ $ | |
| | | @ $ | |
| | | @ $ | |
| | | @ $ | |

Check here to receive our book catalog     ❑          free

**Shipping Costs**

*By Priority Mail: first book $4.50, each additional book $1.00*
*By UPS and to Canada: first book $5.50, each additional book $1.50*
*For rush orders and other countries call us at (510) 865-5282*

TOTAL _____
Less discount @ _____ %        (_____)
TOTAL COST OF BOOKS _____
Calif. residents add sales tax _____
Shipping & handling _____
**TOTAL ENCLOSED** _____
*Please pay in U.S. funds only*

❑ Check  ❑ Money Order  ❑ Visa  ❑ MasterCard  ❑ Discover

Card # _____ Exp. date _____

Signature _____

*Complete and mail to:*
**Hunter House Inc., Publishers**
PO Box 2914, Alameda CA 94501-0914
Website: www.hunterhouse.com
**Orders: (800) 266-5592** or **email: ordering@hunterhouse.com**
Phone (510) 865-5282 Fax (510) 865-4295

IMP3 -- 05/2002